THE ELITE FORCES MANUAL OF
MENTAL & PHYSICAL
ENDURANCE

THE ELITE FORCES MANUAL OF
MENTAL & PHYSICAL ENDURANCE

How to reach your physical and mental peak

Alexander Stilwell

THOMAS DUNNE BOOKS
ST. MARTIN'S GRIFFIN ❧ NEW YORK

THOMAS DUNNE BOOKS
An imprint of St. Martin's Press

www.stmartins.com

Library of Congress Cataloging-in-Publication Data
on file at the Library of Congress

ISBN: 0-312-34818-5

EAN: 978-0-312-34818-2

Editorial and design by
Amber Books Ltd
Bradley's Close
74–77 White Lion Street
London N1 9PF
United Kingdom
www.amberbooks.co.uk

Project Editor: Michael Spilling
Design: Hawes Design
Picture Research: Terry Forshaw
Illustrations: Tony Randell Illustration

Printed in Thailand

10 9 8 7 6 5 4 3

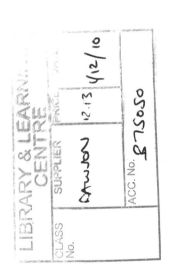

PUBLISHER'S NOTE
Neither the author or the publisher accept responsibility for any loss, injury, or
damage caused as a result of the use of techniques described in this book.
Nor for any prosecutions or proceedings brought or instigated against any person
or body that may result from using these techniques.

CONTENTS

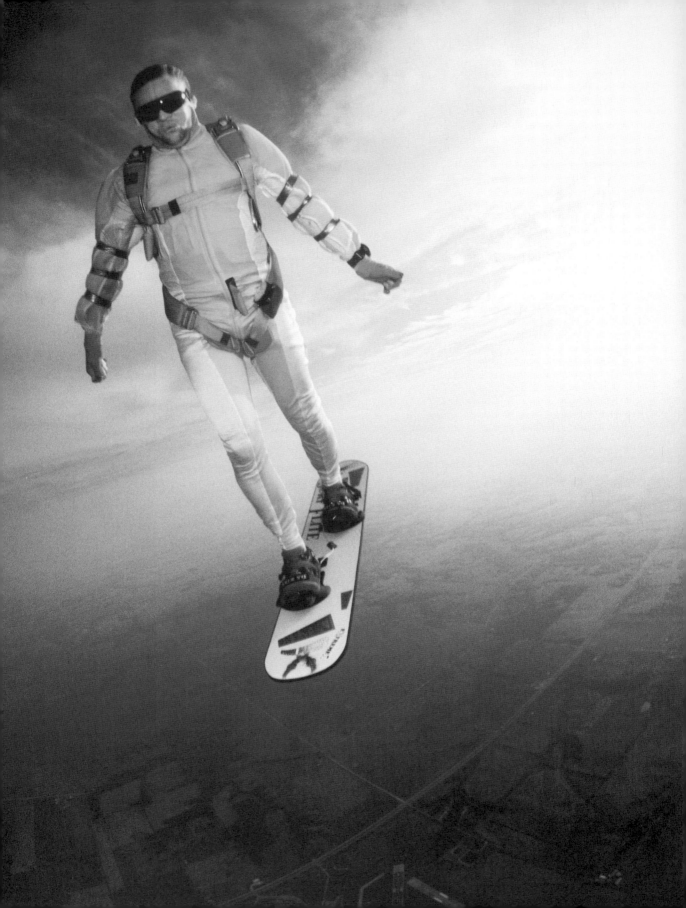

Introduction

'You are what you think' is a well-known phrase but, like many familiar phrases, it deserves closer scrutiny. While the mind controls the physical body in a direct way through the will, the mind itself is divided into the conscious and the subconscious.

The subconscious stores influences that may have been picked up since childhood, and these influences can affect an individual's conscious assessment of their ability to overcome obstacles. Somebody who has had a history of being 'put down' whenever they open their mouth, for example, may have developed an irrational fear of speaking in public. To quote Henry Ford: 'Think you can, think you can't, either way you'll be right.'

Facing Fears

In his book *Call it Courage*, Armstrong Sperry tells the story of a Polynesian boy called Mafatu, who was afraid of the sea. Mafatu means 'Stout Heart' in Polynesian and his name, added to the fact that his island was surrounded by the element he most feared, presented Mafatu with a significant problem. Either he had to accept the name of 'Coward', which he was increasingly called behind his back, and never engage with the source of his fear, or he had to do something about it. Luckily for him, he chose to confront his fear and set out to sea in a small canoe with a couple of pets. By facing his fear and overcoming the challenge, Mafatu was able to return to his island having lived up to his name.

It should be noted that the boy was not named 'Coward' or 'Weakling' at birth. He was given a name that implies high expectations and a certain inherent dignity. The name, however, is also owed to the achievements of his predecessors. Mafatu comes from a long line of 'stout hearts'. It is not, however, enough to 'inherit' courage; he has to prove it to others, and also to himself. In other words, being born of a line of brave people does not exonerate him from having to face fear himself. Courageous

Opposite: The popularity of extreme sports – *sport extrem* in French – demonstrates the fundamental human need to face challenges and overcome them, even if it is necessary for some people to build those challenges themselves.

people, therefore, are not people who have an absence of fear, but they are people who have learned to overcome fear. The experience of overcoming fear in certain circumstances gives them confidence when faced with a similar set of circumstances, although they may still experience the sensation of fear.

Fear of the unknown is natural, but many people populate this unknown with imaginary scenes that are unlikely ever to take place, thus increasing their irrational fear. Note Guardini's words again: 'living means advancing into this unknown region'. In other words, if, like Mafatu, you listen to your fears and do not advance into the unknown region, you are not really living, and you are not living up to either the expectations of others or the expectations conferred upon you by your own dignity as a human being.

Physical and Mental Endurance

Having taken courage into your hands and advanced into the unknown region, whether it be the sea or some other area of challenge, it is not much good to simply get your toes wet and skip out again. The next stage involves staying with it and seeing it through. For Mafatu, like the explorers on the *Kon-Tiki* expedition, he had to encounter storms, dangerous sea animals and other rigours, and endure the journey until it was complete. The journey and all of its challenges helped to build his character and help him to prove that 'Tough times never last, tough people do!' (Robert Schuller)

Many lasting stories of courage imply endurance and tenacity as part of the deal – it is not just a question of turning up and being there, you have to last the course. Usually you only last

Right: The Polynesian boy Mafatu faces the waves. Courage is in proportion to the fear that some challenge arouses in a particular person. Many fears are understandable; others are somewhat irrational. By overcoming the fear, however, courage and confidence are born.

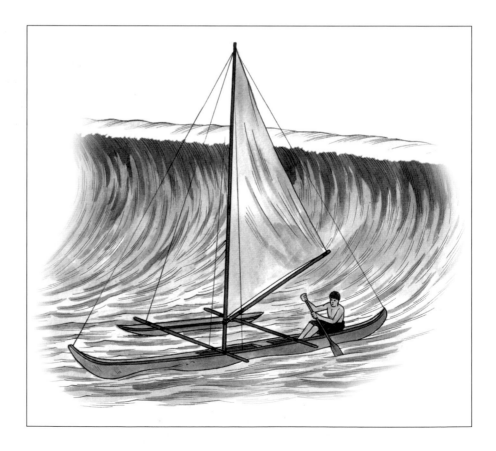

the course if your mental fitness is not only equal, but also superior to your physical fitness. Those people who surpass even this level of achievement, however, have something else: they have the spiritual or subconscious foundations to take them beyond what conscious mental reasoning or grit would deem possible. From those who belong to this hall of fame, everyone will have their favourites. There are the masters of the sea, the intrepid explorers who set out from Portugal and Spain in the fifteenth century to discover the unknown world in which they lived; there are the men and women who have circumnavigated the globe in yachts or other craft, such as Robin Knox Johnston and Emma Richards; and those who have attempted extraordinary journeys to prove a theory, such as Thor Heyerdahl and the men of the *Kon-Tiki* and *Ra* expeditions. There are the masters of the land: men and women who have set off on incredible journeys, such as Marco Polo, or who have scaled mountains with limited equipment or backup. Joining these people are the masters of the air, such as the early pioneers of air mail – Saint-Exupéry, for example.

Masters of the Sea

Ferdinand Magellan led the expedition that first circumnavigated the globe in 1519, his adventure roughly equivalent in those days to a modern journey to Mars. Hot-headed, belligerent and ruthless, Magellan possessed both the drive and determination to carry off such a staggering journey, but he was not a pleasant person. His pride and his thirst for glory made enemies of his own shipmates and of the natives who finally killed him. Although the expedition was successful, Magellan himself did not live to savour the victory.

Captain James Cook was to circumnavigate the globe three times, and his discoveries led to

HAVE COURAGE

Courage has been described as:

'...the confidence required for living with a view to the future, for acting, building, assuming responsibilities, and forming ties. For, in spite of our precautions, the future is in each case the unknown. But living means advancing into this unknown region, which may lie before us like a chaos into which we must venture.'

Roman Guardini

a massive increase in Britain's imperial possessions, including the island continent of Australia. He was also the first man to circumnavigate Antarctica. Like Magellan, Cook lost his life in a scuffle with natives, but his personality was very different to that of the Portuguese man. Cook was taciturn and self-controlled, almost a 'grey man'. He was not the type of person you would want to cross, but he did not let his emotions get the better of him. Strangely enough, a rare fit of anger over the theft of a goat led to his untimely death.

Robin Knox-Johnston was the first man to sail round the world single-handed, which he accomplished in 1969 when he won the Golden Globe Race against nine other contenders, none of whom finished. Knox-Johnston has been quoted as saying, 'Whether you are an amateur or a professional, young or old, there are always new goals and challenges to aspire to in life.'

Knox-Johnston describes the scale of the challenge in his book *A World of My Own*: 'no one knew if a boat could even survive at sea for [...] that distance without support. No one

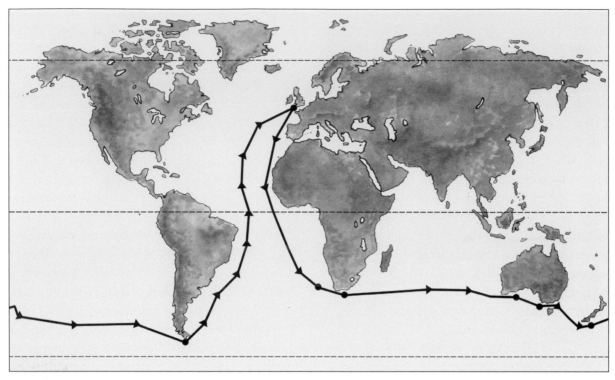

Above: Robin Knox-Johnston was the first man to perform a single-handed circumnavigation of the globe by sea.
He left Falmouth on 14 June 1968, rounded Cape Horn on 17 January 1969 and returned to Falmouth on 22 April 1969.

thought it would be easy, many thought it impossible, but therein lay its intrinsic challenge; real satisfaction comes from achieving something difficult.' Knox-Johnston also writes about the other challenge that faces all men and women – personality: 'It was a distinctive trait in my character that when faced with a problem or job in which I was not at once deeply interested, I would do all I could to avoid tackling it, even to taking on a more difficult, even dangerous task which did hold my interest.'

Emma Richards was only 27 years old when she took part in the 2002–03 Around Alone solo yacht race. Starting in New York on 15 September 2002, she sailed more than 48,000km (30,000 miles) before crossing the finishing line on 4 May 2003, becoming the first British woman and youngest ever competitor to

complete the challenge. Strangely enough, Emma Richards does not enjoy being alone, and she found solo sailing for such long periods soul-destroying. She had to cope not only with being alone, but also with hurricanes and icebergs. She also had to hand-stitch a ripped Kevlar sail on the journey and could snatch only pockets of sleep of about 30 minutes' duration. Emma Richards not only demonstrated remarkable stamina, determination and skill, but she also overcame anyone's worst enemy – the self.

Masters of the Land

Wilfred Thesiger was one of the most famous explorers of Arabia. He made two epic journeys across the Rub 'al Khali, or Empty Quarter, 647,250 square kilometres (250,000 square miles) of desert, with dunes 160km (100 miles) long and 3280m (1000ft) high. This was a place where there was little more than sand, sun and the threat of death either from the environment or from hostile Bedouin.

Thesiger was inspired by the hard life of the Arabs and sought to emulate their ascetic way of life, recognizing that it was hardship that made the desert dwellers such fine people. Thesiger was not a sentimental man: he shot two lion cubs that he had reared because he feared they might grow into man-eaters. He was a war hero who fought for the British in Abyssinia In 1941 and later joined the Special Air Service (SAS) in the Western Desert under David Stirling. For him, hardship was like a magnet. He tested himself against some of the harshest places on the planet and was not found wanting. Known to African tribespeople as Sangalai, 'the old bull elephant who walks by himself', Thesiger found strength in the purity of the desert surroundings. In this way he was similar to the religious hermits and contemplative monks who went into the desert or the mountains to commune with God.

T.E. Lawrence (Lawrence of Arabia) was an expert Arabist who was useful to the British authorities in Cairo, where he helped to draw up maps. The death of both of his brothers on the Western Front spurred him to a more active participation in the war and he helped persuade British authorities that the Arab revolt against the Turks should be actively supported.

After joining Sheikh Faysal, Lawrence began to organize ground-breaking guerrilla hit-and-run operations that were to be copied later by Mao Tse-tung and which have become the foundation of modern special operations.

Right: Wilfred Thesiger, like T.E. Lawrence before him, was drawn by the barren landscapes of the desert and identified profoundly with the simple, hardy Arabs who made their home there.

Lawrence dressed like, and to all intents and purposes became, one of the Arabs; he endured incredible hardships, such as the two-month trek across the desert culminating in the capture of Aqaba. He demonstrated extreme endurance, as well as the ability to devise novel military operations in a hostile environment, and was also able to inspire and lead the Arab tribesmen. Lawrence was ascetic to the point of masochism and his career seems, like the sand dunes he traversed, to be mixed with rapturous peaks followed by painful descents. Although he turned down the signs of public recognition in England, he also wrote the The Seven Pillars of Wisdom, a masterly epic that was to make him a legend.

Robert Falcon Scott was a British naval officer who seems to have shared some of the personality traits of Captain James Cook. He

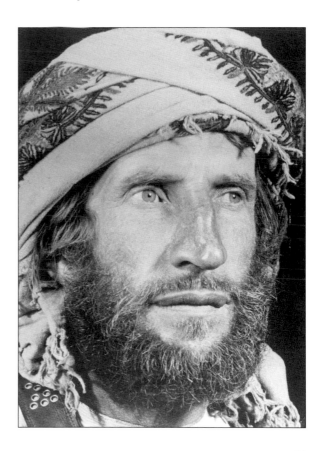

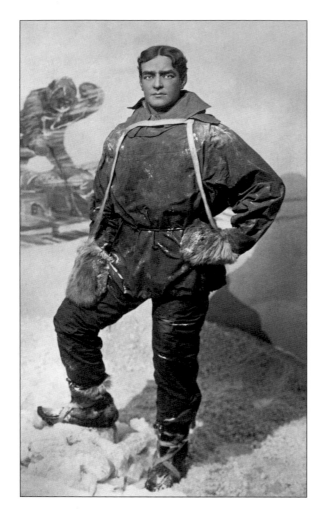

Oates subsequently died. Only 17km (11 miles) from their destination they were confined to their tent by a fierce nine-day blizzard and had no choice but to wait for death. 'Had we lived,' he wrote, 'I should have had a tale to tell of the hardihood, endurance and courage of my companions which would have stirred the heart of every Englishman. These rough notes and our dead bodies must tell the tale.' Amundsen wrote of Scott and his team: 'Bravery, determination, strength, they did not lack.... A little more experience ... would have crowned their work with success.'

Ernest Shackleton travelled with Scott on the British National Antarctic Expedition and later led the British Antarctic (Nimrod) Expedition in 1907, during which he came to within 156km (97 miles) of the South Pole. In 1914, he led the British Imperial Trans-Antarctic Expedition that was to cross Antarctica via the South Pole. The expedition ship *Endurance* was crushed in the pack ice, and Shackleton and five companions made an 1300km (800-mile) journey in a whale boat from Elephant Island to South Georgia to seek help, an incredible feat of seamanship and fortitude. Once at South Georgia, the men had to cross the island, which was a feat in itself, before they reached an aid post. An elaborate rescue operation was then conducted to rescue the rest of *Endurance*'s crew.

Shackleton not only had determination; he was also a meticulous planner who anticipated problems and challenges as far as he could and took steps to circumvent them. Shackleton knew that they could not rely on luck once they were on Elephant Island, that they could not just

was a natural leader and was also a skilled scientific investigator, characteristics that speak of quiet strength. The expedition he led to reach the South Pole in 1910 was fraught with difficulties, bad luck and some planning failures. The motor sledges broke down, the dog teams had to return to base, and the ponies were shot. Scott, along with E.A. Wilson, H.R. Bowers, L.E.G. Oates and Edgar Evans, reached the South Pole on 18 January 1912 after an 81-day trek, only to find that Roald Amundsen had got there a month before them. The men were forced set off on the return journey in increasingly bad weather, and Evans and later wait to be rescued. He studiously planned the trip to South Georgia, and picked his team carefully, taking with him the best navigator in the whole crew, Frank Worsley. By leaving nothing to chance, by carefully preparing the boat and picking the right team, Shackleton raised the chances of success to their highest point, taking into account the adverse circumstances. It was not a gamble that paid off; it was a calculated risk where teamwork, competence and professionalism backed up by toughness won the day.

Ranulph Fiennes is described in the *Guinness Book of Records* as the world's greatest living explorer. He has led more than 30 expeditions, some of the most remarkable of which are the first polar circumnavigation of the world and the first unsupported crossing of the Antarctic continent. An attempt to make the first solo unsupported trek to the North Pole ended in failure when Fiennes suffered severe frostbite after attempting to retrieve a pair of sledges that had fallen through the ice. Fiennes is fully aware of the value of physical fitness in striving to reach your goals and one of his many achievements includes running seven marathons in seven consecutive days in different parts of the world. He is also a proponent of self-motivation and personal determination, as well as the ability to choose the right team for a given task.

Paula Radcliffe has held the record as the world's fastest woman marathon runner. She completed the London Marathon in 2003 in a time of 2:15.25, but success had been hard won. In the early days of her athletics career, Radcliffe was known for her plucky running at the front of the pack, but also for her weakness in the final sprint. As such, she was in danger of becoming a gallant British loser. However, Radcliffe did not enter races to lose. The solution seemed to be to take the sprint to her competitors, not at the end

of the race, as you might expect, but throughout the whole race, so that by the end the competition had no sprint left in them. That was the theory, but it did not always work, as was demonstrated in the 10,000m race at the Sydney Olympics, when two Ethiopians and a Portuguese competitor outstripped her in the final lap.

Radcliffe bounced back and in 2002 set a scorching pace in the Flora London Marathon. She followed this up with first place in the 2002 Commonwealth Games 5000m and in the 2002 European Championships 10,000m. In another Flora London Marathon on 13 April 2003, Paula Radcliffe not only won the race, but also took two minutes off her own world record, a performance described in the *Glasgow Herald* as 'the most stunning endurance performance in history, male or female'. The run was described by Peter Matthews, an expert on long-distance running, as 'simply the greatest achievement in the history of the sport'.

By 2004, such was Paula Radcliffe's reputation that she arrived in Athens for the Olympics with a gold medal effectively reserved. It was, however, not to be. In one of the most dramatic scenes in the history of the Marathon, Paula Radcliffe, worn down by heat and an opposition that refused to be broken by her searing pace, gave up. She also stopped before the finish of the 10,000m.

Marathons are nothing if not about endurance, determination and staying the course, and for someone as dedicated and hard-working as Paula Radcliffe, the impact of the failure was all the greater. For someone as determined as Paula Radcliffe, however, there could be only one solution. On 7 November 2004, she competed in and won the New York Marathon after one of the hardest-fought marathon races ever seen. Radcliffe, who supposedly does not have a sprint finish, outsprinted Susan Chepkemei of Kenya to take the race. It was a remarkable display of staying power and determination.

Paula Radcliffe demonstrates that winners are people who are dedicated to what they do best and who keep on trying. Even after they have supposedly 'given up', they get up and have another go. She is a testament to the saying that 'a quitter never wins and a winner never quits'.

Chris Ryan was a member of B Squadron, 22 Special Air Service Regiment, who were tasked with observing and reporting on the infamous 'Scud' missiles deployed by Iraq during the 1990–91 Gulf War. Ryan, along with the rest of his troop, was dropped in a featureless desert that turned out to be somewhat different from the sandy desert they had trained in. It was as hard as rock, with little by way of cover, and whipped by a searingly cold wind. To make matters worse, they found that they had been dropped within only a few hundred yards of an Iraqi anti-aircraft battery. Compromised by a shepherd boy, they soon found themselves in a firefight with a truckload of Iraqi soldiers and having to run for their lives. With little choice other than to ditch their 45kg (100lb) bergens, they were left to face the rigours of the desert with inadequate clothing and little food or water. As parts of the team lost contact with each other or succumbed to the cold, Ryan soon found

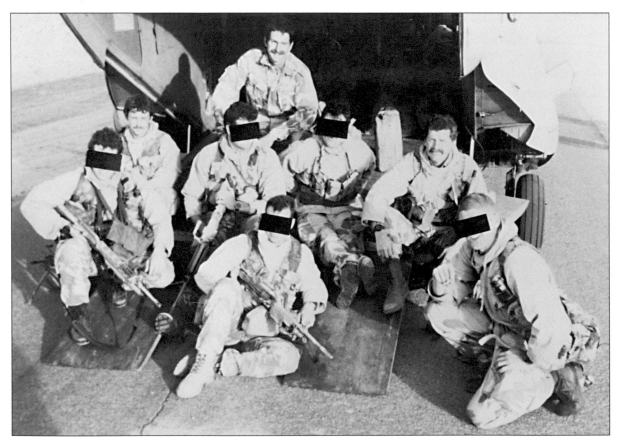

Above: Members of the SAS team, call sign Bravo Two Zero, pose before a Chinook helicopter prior to departure on their ill-fated mission. Chris Ryan is on the far left. Three died; four were captured; one got away.

himself on his own. Pacing across the desert at night, powered by sheer determination, he was being followed by two Iraqi army vehicles. If this had been a normal soldier from a normal regiment, the result would have been inevitable – either death or capture. Unfortunately for the Iraqis, however, they were chasing a soldier from the world's premier special forces regiment. Using a disposable US hand-held tank missile, Ryan destroyed first one vehicle, then the other. None of the Iraqis survived the encounter.

Ryan plunged on into the night, sustained by Standard Operating Procedures (SOPs) and a rugged morale. He endured freezing days and nights, blistering feet and all the effects of inadequate nutrition and hydration. Eventually, he crossed the border into a neutral but unfriendly Syria, his mind and body scarred by the experience. Three of his colleagues had been killed, and four had been captured.

The fate of Bravo Two Zero is somewhat reminiscent, in microcosm, of the ill-fated Operation Market Garden at the end of World War II, when crack British paratroopers were let down by faulty radios and other organizational failures. The SAS troop had been given the wrong radio frequencies and aged maps, and the appreciation of the ground and the weather conditions was astonishingly faulty. Failure to anticipate the freezing conditions of the Iraqi winter meant that essential warm clothing was left behind. Equipment overloads meant that even the warm kit they had was discarded in favour of essential operational equipment. Anxiety about the enemy caused Ryan to replace essential nutritional supplies in his belt kit with ammunition.

The story of Bravo Two Zero reveals how even the mostly highly trained soldiers can be compromised by bad organization. Chris Ryan revealed that the calibre of an SAS soldier is

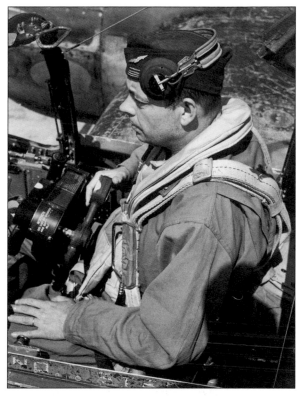

Above: Antoine de Saint-Exupéry (1900–44), a pioneer aviator, flew perilous journeys over the Andes and the North African desert. He lyrically transposed his adventures into a number of classic books.

such that he could overcome not only the enemy and the forces of nature, but also abandonment by his own regiment.

Masters of the Air

Antoine de Saint-Exupéry was a pioneering pilot, writer and poet who to helped set up some of the first mail routes across the Sahara desert and across the Andes mountains. He had several plane accidents, the worst being in the Libyan desert in 1936, and he was constantly faced with the possibility of death as he battled in rudimentary aircraft over massive deserts and mountains, and against the overwhelming forces of the elements. Eventually death caught up with him, though he was not killed by nature, but by his fellow men when he was shot down on a reconnaissance flight in North Africa in 1943.

Saint-Exupéry was not so much an extraordinary man as he was an ordinary man who did extraordinary things. Like many of the great adventurers, he was attracted to simplicity, and he also had a strong sense of duty.

Captain Scott O'Grady proved that a master of the air also needs to know how to master the land. Flying over Bosnia with a wingman on 2 June 1995 while enforcing a no-fly zone over the Former Republic of Yugoslavia, the two planes were tracked by a Serb surface-to-air missile (SAM) unit that had been positioned south of Banja Luka. The Serbs switched the missile tracking system on and off in order to conceal its position from the Allied forces. Confident that

RISK TAKING

Saint-Exupéry was aware of the risks that he took, and he was also aware that many people live their entire lives without facing risks and therefore never discover their true capabilities.

'Self-discovery comes when man measures himself against an obstacle,' he wrote, and, 'A sense of vocation helps man to liberate himself, certainly; but it is just as necessary to liberate the vocation. Nights in the air, nights in the desert ... these are rare opportunities, offered to few men. And yet, when circumstances bring them to life, all men reveal the same needs.'

Wind, Sand and Stars,
Antoine de Saint-Exupéry

there was no unwarranted threat in the area, the two US F-16s were not accompanied by electronic jamming aircraft or by planes armed with HARM anti-radiation missiles that could lock on to a missile battery radar.

When warning signals came up on his instrument panel, O'Grady knew a missile was chasing him. Unfortunately, as he was flying in cloud, he could make no visual contact in order to take evasive action. One missile exploded between the two planes; the other hit O'Grady's F-16 flat in the belly. As the plane began to break up, O'Grady pulled his ejection-seat lever and blew out of the cockpit.

He landed safely in a clearing and headed immediately for a nearby woods, where he kept his head down. A man and a boy wondered by at one point and he saw armed men in the distance, but he remained still, like a hunted animal. Once the immediate danger had passed, O'Grady organized his sleeping arrangements, covering himself with hessian during the day and only moving at night to catch insects or eat grass for minimum nutrition. He took care not to send out a radio signal too soon, as he knew the Serbs would be listening in to pinpoint his position, but on the fourth day O'Grady signalled his location and on the fifth day spoke into his radio. Aboard USS *Kearsage*, O'Grady's home aircraft carrier, the rescue mission was activated.

Conducted in daylight, the rescue mission involved 40 aircraft. Two Cobra helicopters of the 24th Marine Expeditionary Unit came in low and landed in Grady's location, where he had set off a flare at the last minute. Marines from one helicopter secured the perimeter, while Grady ran on to the second.

Despite the considerable air power at their disposal, the danger was far from over. Soon Serb ground units began to engage the helicopters with hand-held missile launchers

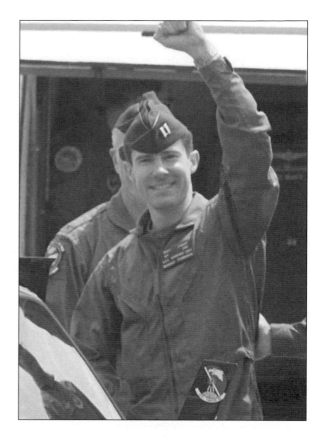

and small arms. The Marines heard the rounds clattering against the fuselage as the aircraft flew onwards. US fighter pilots reported that a Serb missile unit was scanning the area, but they were not given permission to destroy it. Within half an hour, the helicopters were over the sea. Mission accomplished.

Scott O'Grady showed courage and presence of mind. He used his survival training to good effect, and he was determined not to have to use another part of his training for real – resistance to interrogation, which may have involved torture.

From his own account, Scott O'Grady not only came to fully appreciate his own physical freedom, but also came to appreciate what was truly worthwhile in life, namely faith in God and the love of family and friends. Given unexpected time to reflect with his life in danger, for him success and possessions came a poor second to a life dedicated to the service of others.

Masters of Space

Captain James Lovell commanded the third United States lunar attempt, which lifted off on 11 April 1970. At this time, Lovell had travelled more miles than any person in history and, with that amount of experience, a journey to the moon was as close to routine as such a voyage could get. However, two days, seven hours and 54 minutes into the mission, things began to go wrong. There was a loud bang during a routine check, and a red light came on the warning panel called Main B. Lovell's inaccurate phrase said it all: 'Houston, we've had a problem.' Unfortunately, they had not 'had' a problem – the problem was there to stay.

As the electrical specialist Fred Haise headed into the command module, *Odyssey*, more warning lights were coming on. The tunnel running between the lunar module *Aquarius* and the *Odyssey* was pinging under the strain, and voltage readings were almost nonexistent. The chemical powerplants that produced electricity from a reaction between hydrogen and oxygen were not functioning properly. Soon there were so many malfunctions that they had gone beyond every worst-case scenario thrown at them in training.

While the others worked along with Houston through the maze of possible options, Lovell suddenly realized what the problem was as he looked out of the window. There was a large spume of gas coming out from the side of *Odyssey*. An electrical short had exploded

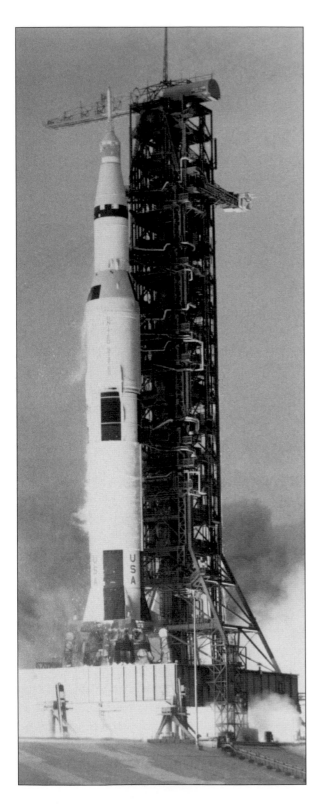

number 2 oxygen tank and the other tank was rapidly emptying. Not only were they not going to land on the moon, but also it was looking doubtful that they would ever land back on earth – the spacecraft was 322,000km (200,000 miles) from earth and heading very rapidly in the wrong direction.

Teams on the ground continued to work furiously round the clock to solve the problem, and Lovell performed feats of mental gymnastics to align *Odyssey* with the stars so that they could alter the craft's trajectory, which on current settings meant they would miss the earth on the return journey by 72,400km (45,000 miles). Lovell then had to orient the spacecraft with the earth, which involved a delicate manouevre using a modified gunsight. His task was to get the horns of the earth's crescent to sit on the crosshairs, then fire up the engine for 14 seconds – known as a burn. Apart from these moments of high adrenalin, there were large blocks of time when they could do little more than wait in extremely cold temperatures and a cramped environment. It was too cold to sleep comfortably. Largely due to Lovell's leadership and example, however, no one lost their temper.

As the craft continued to hurtle towards the earth, tiredness began to take its toll, as well as dehydration. The astronauts had to keep themselves to minimum water rations, like men crossing a desert, and this compounded the negative effect on their concentration. Fortunately, the systems in the craft, which had been closed down to preserve power, restarted perfectly at the vital moment. If the craft's heat shield was undamaged and could cope with the

Left: *Apollo 13* **launches on 11 April 1970. The mission was intended to put men on the moon for the third time; however, the real achievement turned out to be getting those men back to earth safely.**

massive heat of re-entry, they would be OK. And so it was. Soon the *Odyssey* had splashed down and the astronauts were being feted on board an aircraft carrier in the balmy waters of the Pacific.

The *Apollo 13* mission required physical and mental endurance of a high order. Although different in many respects from other, earth-bound journeys, the technical accuracy and nerve required of the crew have parallels with the journey performed by Shackleton and his crew to South Georgia. The space journey demanded intense concentration and patience in a cramped space, while the necessary privations gnawed away at physical and mental faculties. It also required attention to detail of a very high order, for the slightest error in calculation could have sent the craft on an irretrievable course past the earth and into endless orbit. Stuck in their cold craft, the astronauts of *Apollo 13* might have wished to change places with an athlete on a gruelling marathon, where at least they would have had both feet on the ground.

The remarkable fact about these stories is that many of them involve a large element of failure. The 'success' was not so much in achieving the goal, but in overcoming unforeseen obstacles or accidents and getting back despite the odds. However carefully we

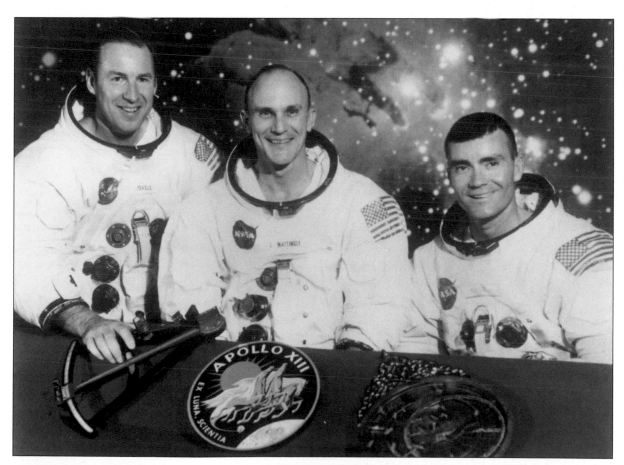

Above: James Lovell, John Young and Fred Haise after their return from the aborted *Apollo 13* mission. The sextant held by Lovell underlines the crucial importance of the correct navigational trajectory on the return flight.

may set our sights on some goal, therefore, the real tests may be totally unpredictable and unforeseen, and it is these that may truly test our character, even more in fact than achieving the original goal. Confidence and success, therefore, may not come so much from 'winning' as from endurance and the journey into our own physical and mental resources. Nevertheless, we must expect success with confidence and be willing for it to occur, and try our best to expect and be prepared for the unexpected.

Decide on Your Goal

You are not likely to reach the South Pole if you have half a mind to reaching the North Pole. You are not likely to land on the moon if your real desire is actually to land on Mars. In short, the more decided that you can be about your goal, the more likely it is that you will achieve it.

The talent that enables sportsmen such as footballer David Beckham to kick a ball in an unstoppable arc into the corner of a net or basketballer Michael Jordan to score from the free-throw line is difficult to quantify. What can be understood, however, is the hours of patient practice that have taken place in training before the critical event – the single-minded determination to be the best and to keep kicking or throwing until it becomes almost second nature. The constant training empowers the mind and the body to perform to their maximum potential when the pressure is on, and for sheer inspiration to do the rest.

To decide on a goal may seem like the easy part, but for many people it is not. To decide on one goal may mean discarding many others, all of which hold their own potential, and therefore it can be a painful and difficult thing to do. Great achievers, however, demonstrate a single-minded ability to focus on their goals, and once the decision has been made obstacles seem to fall before the force of their determination.

REALISTIC GOALS

It is all very well saying you are going to achieve something, but you have to ask yourself whether or not the goal is realistic. The South Pole may be too far for you; the summit of Everest too high. If you set an ambitious and ultimately unachievable goal, the results will be negative and will damage your confidence. It is better to set realistic goals, or staging posts on the way to achieving a larger goal.

Someone relatively unfit and inexperienced who decides to take up running may have been inspired by watching a marathon, but they would be unwise to make the attempt before they have worked through shorter distances. It is no use saying you are going to run a marathon if you cannot run a half-marathon or even an 8km (5-mile) race. By gradually building up ever greater distances, however, an unfit person who can barely run three kilometres (two miles) can indeed achieve the ultimate goal of running 42km (26 miles).

By setting intermediate goals and focusing exclusively on achieving them, an oversized goal can be made manageable. This approach has the added benefit of building your confidence. By using this technique, you can overcome the negative effects of an oversized goal, which can seem overwhelming when viewed in its entirety.

Right: Michael Jordan poised to shoot a goal. Focus, concentration and practice can meld together to produce inspirational results.

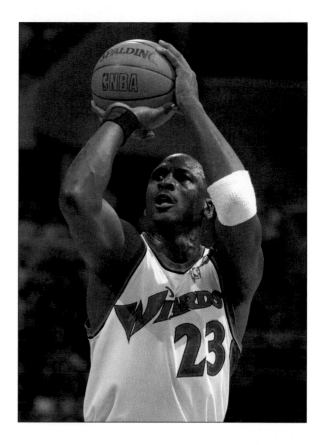

Somebody who carries an alternative option in their backpack, on the other hand, is more likely to turn away from their first choice of goal when the going gets tough. Successful people are sometimes deviated from their goal by *force majeure*, as we have seen, but that is a different story. Setting a goal is not dissimilar to Lovell taking a setting from the sun and targeting the earth on *Apollo 13*. Once that was done, although they could not exactly sit back and enjoy the ride, the astronauts were at least on course and could focus on other peripheral demands. Once the course has been set, things have an uncanny way of falling into place. This is because both consciously and subconsciously we make decisions and use opportunities to attain the goal. This can only happen, however, if the goal is set.

Focus

Focus essentially means the concentration of all your mental and physical powers on a particular event or task. Focus and concentration, therefore, are often the basic ingredients of achievement. Isaac Newton spoke of focus and concentration in the following terms: 'I keep the subject continually before me and wait till the first dawnings open slowly, little by little, into full clear light.' If Isaac Newton had had other things on his mind, then the laws of gravitation, as well as many other scientific discoveries, may have eluded him. The opposite of focus is distraction, which can be brought on by a whole host of worries and preoccupations. However complex the human mind, it is surprisingly ill adept at focusing on two things at once. So if the mind is churning over a problem or distracted by some worry, its ability to properly carry out the task in hand is impaired.

One aid to focus is getting into the habit of living in the present. Distracting worries are often caused by regrets about the past or forebodings about the future. To achieve focus you need to forget about the past (you cannot do anything about it anyway) and take care not to anticipate the future. The future will come, but in the form of each successive present moment. If each of those present moments is being dealt with effectively, with full concentration, then the future is likely to turn out better than it would if our minds were elsewhere.

The mind's ability to focus can be enhanced through training. Certain forms of meditation are a good way to achieve this, as meditation involves clearing the mind of distractions and focusing on a particular word or mantra. At the beginning, the mind is likely to be beset by distractions. It is good practice to acknowledge the distractions, without arguing over them, and then to refocus on the particular word, phrase or visualization. Gradually the 'muscles' of the mind will be strengthened and the distractions in subsequent sessions become less frequent. If meditation is performed regularly, the mind should be clearer and easier to focus during day-to-day activities and when called upon to perform exceptional tasks.

A good example of the ability to focus intently with full concentration is found in the story of James Lovell in *Apollo 13*. Here was an astronaut several thousand miles from earth in a spacecraft that had effectively blown up. In these highly stressful circumstances, and with other astronauts floating around him, Lovell was required to carry out complex mathematical calculations, as well as having to steer the craft within minute degrees of accuracy.

Focus, therefore, is really about living fully in the present moment and not allowing other considerations – for example, other people's performances, expectations or jealousies – to interfere with what you are doing. It is about you and the task or duty of the present moment. Following the principle that the mind cannot focus on two things simultaneously, if your mind is engaged on the task in hand it will be unable to deal with the distracting worries. Anxiety and worry are best dispelled by simply getting on with what needs to be done and, as progress is made, that very progress tends to disprove the discouraging worry.

Commitment

You have set a goal, along with intermediate stages along the way that take into account the realities of the present. In other words, you are not just dreaming about this goal; you are buying yourself a new pair of trainers, ordering books from the library, writing a certain number of words on a page or whatever fits in with your particular goals. You are also focused on what you are doing. You have not allowed distracting worries to hinder you, and you have not allowed the size of the goal to overwhelm you. What you have done today will, when added up, make your ultimate goal achievable.

Something, however, is not quite right. You are going through the motions and keeping to the rules you have set for yourself, but it all seems rather mechanical and uninspiring. If these symptoms occur it can be due to a number of factors. The first is that you have forgotten to rest. It is all very well setting yourself a rigorous schedule and having the self-discipline to keep to it, but having worked long hours into the night and got up early in the morning to start again, a feeling of drag begins to set in. It no longer seems quite as exciting as when you bought that new equipment or read those exciting books. Without rest, your mind and body lose the freshness and vitality that are necessary to produce its best performance. They will come along under orders from your will, but they are dragging their feet.

Building in rest and recreation is an essential part of your goal setting and trying to get round this is counterproductive because, although you may be putting in the hours, you are probably not working as well as you would if you had had some rest, and you are probably less inspired to think up new angles and solutions. If your goal is athletic, rest and recreation may include reading an absorbing book. If your goal is academic and keeps you at your desk, rest and recreation for your mind may mean going out for a long trail run or a walk. Either way, body and mind are given a break from regular activity.

If you have built in proper rest periods and things still seem rather uninspiring, it may mean that there is something wrong with your goal. What you imagined would be a valuable target is somehow not inspiring you. If this is the case, you probably need to sit down and re-examine what really motivates you. There are many ways you can do this, including the use of self-assessment psychometric tests.

Your commitment to your goal will be influenced by the level of its real importance to you. In other words, your motivation will be influenced by the importance of the goal. Commitment and focus are intimately related for, when obstacles arise, as they surely will, whether you choose to go round, over or through them, your determination will be influenced by the importance that the goal holds for you. This commitment to the goal and the satisfaction of reaching it will work differently for different people. For one person it may mean standing on the winner's podium with a gold medal round his or her neck; for another it may mean receiving a cherished regimental green, fawn or red beret; for another it may mean standing unnoticed in a crowd, knowing that they have contributed their little bit to a team effort. Whatever it is, you will know it, and the glow of satisfaction will come from having done your best with your available talents, remaining true to your ideals.

Arguably, the commitment test should come near the beginning of the list, but perhaps it is better to choose your goals without too much thought, then test your commitment to them. You will soon discover whether or not the goals are meaningful or not. Causes of empty goals, or those for which you do not have genuine commitment, can include advice from someone who does not really know your real strengths and talents; the desire to conform; the need to prove something to someone else; or the need to make up for a low opinion of yourself.

Real and lasting commitment will be born of true self-knowledge: the ability to go the way you believe is right no matter what anyone else thinks, the ability to control circumstances rather than letting them control you, a healthy individuality and a recognition of your uniqueness and of your unique talents.

To summarize, you need to select realistic goals, focus on them and commit to them so that you can follow them wholeheartedly. Once you are committed to a goal, everything else should follow. To set out after a goal is like setting out on a journey: you need to plan what you will need on the journey and you also need to analyse your strengths and weaknesses, both mental and physical, to ensure that you will be able to complete the adventure.

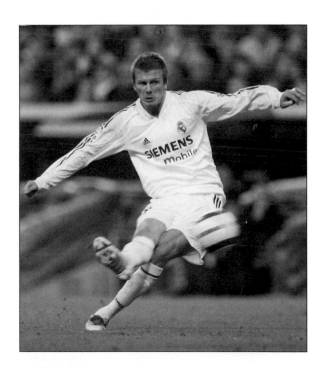

Right: English footballer David Beckham – miraculous shots delivered at key moments of a match seem like inspiration, but are largely the fruit of constant practice.

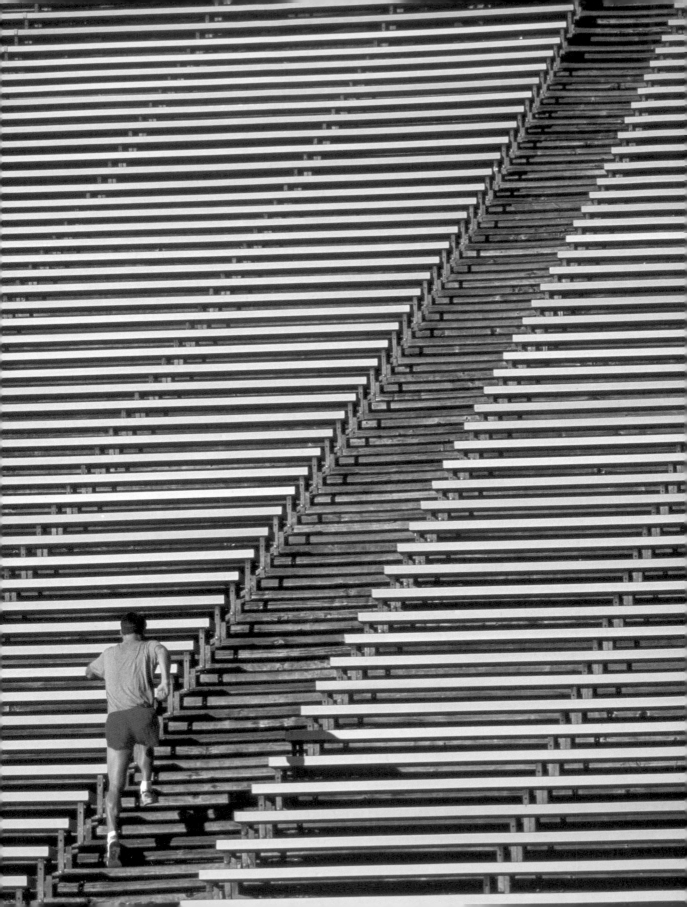

CHAPTER ONE

Physical Preparation

Preparing your body physically is vital to your success in overcoming challenges and reaching goals. You must be in as peak a physical condition as possible to withstand both the physical and mental rigours you will encounter.

When you start a serious and consistent training programme, your body begins to transform itself in various ways. Your bones will start to thicken in your feet and legs and become more robust; your circulation will improve; the walls of the heart thicken and its chambers increase in size; your joints are lubricated and work more efficiently; the muscles in the diaphragm become stronger and more efficient, which aids breathing; the number of blood vessels that supply each muscle cell is increased and the mitochondria multiply, enhancing the cell's use of oxygen to produce energy. The rate at which the cell burns fat to produce energy is also increased. Overall, the fast-twitch muscles in your body increase their resistance to fatigue. The respiratory system is cleared of mucus while running, which enables you to breathe more clearly. The skin becomes more efficient in regulating heat and resisting cold, and more efficient perspiration tends to have a cleansing effect that reduces the likelihood of catching skin-related infections.

Your body's natural reaction to exercise training is to prepare itself for an even bigger task next time. It is as if the body that has been

Opposite: Resistance training of any kind helps to build muscle and strength. Running up a series of steps is an excellent form of resistance training, as well as providing a tough cardiovascular workout.

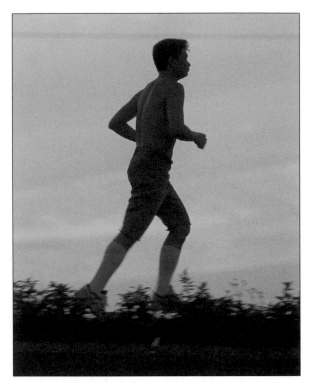

Above: Men and women were born to run; it is in our genes. The physical and mental benefits of a consistent running programme cannot be overemphasized.

Health Check

Before you set off towards your goal, it is vital to take an inventory on where you stand now in the physical department, otherwise you are likely to do yourself damage. You also need to analyse your habits, such as what you eat and drink, and how much of your time is sedentary or active.

Resting Heart Rate

A rapid way of assessing your overall fitness is literally to take your pulse and assess your resting heart rate (RHR). A slow, regular pulse is the sign of a fit person, while a fast, erratic pulse is a sign of someone who is unfit. Even if your pulse is reasonably steady when you measure it while resting, you also need to be aware of what it is like after you have exerted yourself.

A strong, healthy heart pumps blood round the body in a regular, measured way and it is well able to adjust to the extra strains placed upon it by physical as well as emotional exertion. An unfit heart has to beat more rapidly to get the necessary quantity of blood round the body, and under the strain of physical or emotional exertion it beats even more rapidly. One way of visualizing this is to imagine the speedometer and rev counter in a car. In a fit person, the speedometer can be taken to a high speed with the rev counter remaining comfortably within the 'black zone'. In an unfit person, the rev indicator veers quickly into the 'red zone' when high speed is attempted.

You can test your pulse at rest either by counting it for a minute or by counting it for 10 seconds and multiplying by six. If you are in good condition, your pulse rate will probably be around 60 bpm (beats per minute). If you are seriously fit, the score may be as low as 40 or 50 bpm. The average person will probably score about 80 bpm, while scores of 90 to 100 bpm show decreasing levels of fitness. Women need

trained to full capacity uses the following logic: that was too close for comfort, so I will increase my capacity to make it more manageable next time, and prepare for an even bigger load.

The starting point for a fitness training programme, if you are relatively unfit at the outset, is low-intensity training that focuses on aerobic activity as well as strengthening the essential muscles of the body, such as the leg, back, stomach and abdominal muscles. If you are planning to join a military training programme, there is likely to be a large disparity between your current level of fitness and the level of fitness that you will have achieved by the time you graduate from the course. The fitter you are on arrival, the less stressful and painful the experience is likely to be.

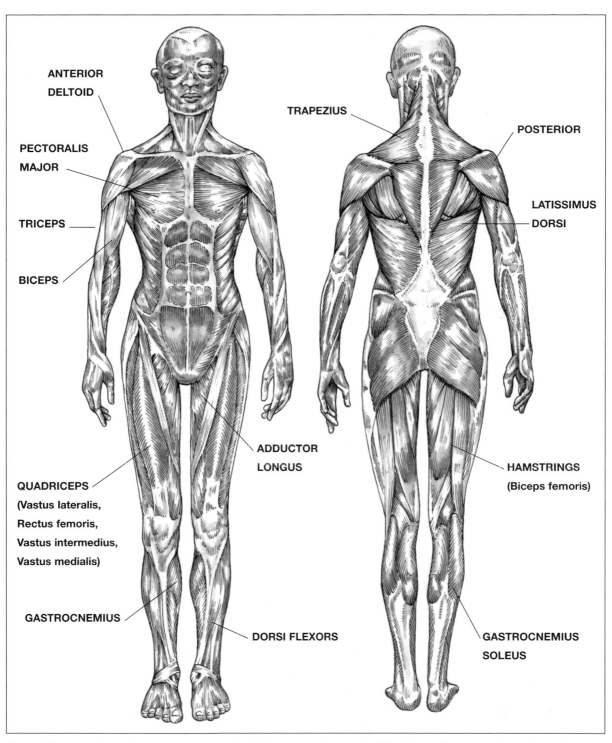

ANTERIOR
DELTOID

PECTORALIS
MAJOR

TRICEPS

BICEPS

TRAPEZIUS

POSTERIOR

LATISSIMUS
DORSI

ADDUCTOR
LONGUS

QUADRICEPS
(Vastus lateralis,
Rectus femoris,
Vastus intermedius,
Vastus medialis)

GASTROCNEMIUS

DORSI FLEXORS

HAMSTRINGS
(Biceps femoris)

GASTROCNEMIUS
SOLEUS

Above: The muscular make-up of the human body is extremely complex. The above diagram outlines the main muslces and muscle groups.

US Marine Corps Preparation Training Schedule

WEEK	MON	TUES	WED	THUR	FRI	SAT	SUN
1	3km (2-mile) run (SLOW STEADY) • Push-ups 3 sets of 10 • Pull-ups 3 sets of 3 • Flexed-arm hang 20 secs x 3 • Sit-ups 3 sets of 20 • Tricep dips 3 sets of 15 • Bend & thrust 10/10	0.6km (1-mile) interval sprints	• Push-ups 3 sets of 10 • Pull-ups (MAX OR 20) • Flexed-arm hang (MAX OR 70 sec) • Sit-ups 3 sets of 20 • Tricep dips 3 sets of 15 • Bend & thrust 10/10/10	REST	60 minutes of cross training • Push-ups 3 sets of 10 • Pull-ups 3 sets of 3 • Flexed-arm hang 20 secs x 3 • Sit-ups (MAX OR 100) • Tricep dips 3 sets of 15 • Bend & thrust 15/10/10	5km (3-mile) run TIMED	REST
2	4km (2½-mile) run (STEADY) • Push-ups 3 sets of 15 • Pull-ups (MAX OR 20) • Flexed-arm hang (MAX OR 70 SEC) • Sit-ups 3 sets of 25 • Tricep dips 3 sets of 15 • Bend & Thrust 15/10/10	4km (2½-mile) run TEMPO/CHANGE PACE	REST	0.6km (1-mile) interval sprints	60 minutes of cross training • Push-ups 3 sets of 15 • Pull-ups 3 sets of 3 • Flexed-arm hang 30 secs x 3 • Sit-ups (MAX OR 100) • Tricep dips 3 sets of 15 • Bend & thrust 15/15/10	4km (2½-mile) run MATCH 5km (3-mile) PACE, EASE DOWN LAST MILE	REST
3	4km (2½-mile) run (SLOW STEADY) • Push-ups (MAX OR 50) • Pull-ups 3 sets of 5 • Flexed-arm hang 30 secs x 3 • Sit-ups 3 sets of 25 • Tricep dips 3 sets of 20 • Bend & thrust 15/15/10	2km (1¼-mile) run in boots (STEADY STATE)	• Push-ups 3 sets of 20 • Pull-ups (MAX OR 20) • Flexed-arm hang (MAX OR 70 SEC) • Sit-ups 3 sets of 25 • Tricep dips 3 sets of 20 • Bend & thrust 15/15/15	2km (1¼-mile) interval sprints	60 minutes of cross training • Push-ups 3 sets of 20 • Pull-ups 3 sets of 5 • Flexed-arm hang 30 secs x 3 • Sit-ups (MAX OR 100) • Tricep dips 3 sets of 20 • Bend & thrust 15/15/15	5km (3-mile) run TIMED	REST
4	8km (5-mile) run (STEADY) • Push-ups 3 sets of 20 • Pull-ups (MAX OR 20) • Flexed-arm hang (MAX OR 70 SEC) • Sit-ups 3 sets of 30 • Tricep dips 3 sets of 20 • Bend & thrust 20/15/15	3km (2-mile) run in boots	• Push-ups (MAX OR 60) • Pull-ups 3 sets of 5 • Flexed-arm hang 40 secs x 3 • Sit-ups 3 sets of 30 • Tricep dips 3 sets of 20 • Bend & thrust 20/15/15	3km (2-mile) interval sprints	60 minutes of cross training • Push-ups 3 sets of 20 • Pull-ups 3 sets of 5 • Flexed-arm hang 40 secs x 3 • Sit-ups (MAX OR 100) • Tricep dips 3 sets of 20 • Bend & thrust 20/20/15	6km (4-mile) run	REST

US Marine Corps Preparation Training Schedule

WEEK	MON	TUES	WED	THUR	FRI	SAT	SUN
5	3km (2-mile) run in boots	10km (6-mile) run SLOW STEADY • Push-ups (1 SET TO MAX OR 60) • Pull-ups 3 sets of 8 • Flexed-arm hang 45 secs x 3 • Sit-ups 3 sets of 40 • Tricep dips 3 sets of 25 • Bend & thrust 20/20/15	• Push-ups 3 sets of 25 • Pull-ups (1 SET TO MAX OR 20) • Flexed-arm hang (1 SET TO MAX OR 70 SEC) • Sit-ups 3 sets of 40 • Tricep dips 3 sets of 25	5km (3-mile) run for PFT time	60 minutes of cross training • Push-ups 3 sets of 25 • Pull-ups 3 sets of 8 • Flexed-arm hang 45 secs x 3 • Sit-ups (1 SET TO MAX OR 100 INSIDE 2 MINS) • Tricep dips 3 sets of 25 • Bend & thrust 20/20/20	6km (4-mile) run STRONG TEMPO	REST
6	8km (5-mile) run TEMPO • Push-ups (1 SET TO MAX OR 65) • Pull-ups 3 sets to fatigue • Flexed-arm hang 3 sets to fatigue • Sit-ups 3 sets to fatigue • Tricep dips 3 sets of 30 • Bend & thrust 20/20/20	3km (2-mile) run in boots	• Push-ups 3 sets of 30 • Pull-ups 3 sets to fatigue • Flexed-arm hang 3 sets to fatigue • Sit-ups 3 sets to fatigue • Tricep dips 3 sets of 30 • Bend & thrust 25/20/20	5km (3-mile) run STEADY	60 minutes of cross training • Push-ups 1 SET MAXIMUM REPS • Pull-ups 3 sets to fatigue • Flexed-arm hang 3 sets to fatigue • Sit-ups 3 sets to fatigue • Tricep dips 3 sets of 30 • Bend & thrust 25/20/20	11km (7-mile) run SLOW STEADY	REST
7	5km (3-mile) run FOR TIME • Push-ups 3 sets of 30 • Pull-ups 1 SET TO MAX • Flexed-arm hang 1 SET TO MAX POS SECS • Sit-ups 3 sets to fatigue • Tricep dips 3 sets of 35 • Bend & thrust 25/25/20	5km (3-mile) run in boots	REST	6km (4-mile) run STEADY	60 minutes of cross training • Push-ups 3 sets of 30 • Pull-ups 3 sets to fatigue • Flexed-arm hang 3 sets to fatigue • Sit-ups (MAX IN 2 MIN) • Tricep dips 3 sets of 35 • Bend & thrust 25/25/20	10km (6-mile) run TEMPO/CHANGE	REST
8	5km (3-mile) run STRONG/TEMPO • Push-ups 3 sets of 30 • Pull-ups 3 sets to fatigue • Flexed-arm hang 3 sets to fatigue • Sit-ups 3 sets to fatigue • Tricep dips 3 sets of 40 • Bend & thrust 20/20/20	3km (2-mile) run in boots	• Push-ups 3 sets of 30 • Pull-ups 3 sets to fatigue • Flexed-arm hang 3 sets to fatigue • Sit-ups 3 sets to fatigue • Tricep dips 3 sets of 40	6km (4-mile) run TEMPO	60 minutes of cross training • Push-ups 3 sets of 30 • Pull-ups 1 max set • Flexed-arm hang 70 sec max • Sit-ups 1 max set • Tricep dips 3 sets of 40 • Bend & thrust 20/20/20	REST	REST

LEGEND/DESCRIPTER
SLOW STEADY — maintenance of a pace which would still allow the ability to converse with a training partner or colleague.
STEADY — selection of a pace that is quicker than slow steady and can still be maintained over a stated distance. Individual will be breathing heavy but controlled.
TEMPO — variation of pace throughout the run, selection of periods of sustained open-pace running interspersed with more moderate recovery running, selecting various terrain or surface.
STRONG TEMPO — As above with longer more sustained periods or legs of open-running higher-intensity effort intermittent with lighter recovery/steady running.
TIMED — strong best-effort run, to provide periodic individual objective markers to monitor progress and use data for realistic goal setting for future aims or events.

to take into account the fact that their hearts tend to beat about 5 bpm faster than men's.

Heart rate can be affected by other factors. If you are slightly ill, with a cold or sore throat, your heartbeat may be raised. Tiredness can also cause a raised heartbeat, as can stress and anxiety. Certain kinds of stimulants, such as coffee or tea, can increase your heart rate.

Training Heart Rate

Your training heart rate (THR) gives an indication of how your heart reacts under exertion, and this in turn gives a good picture of your fitness. As with your RHR, however, various factors can influence the result, such as tiredness or overtraining. Your

THR is the rate at which your heart beats to provide optimum cardiovascular training and conditioning. The THR lies between 70 and 80 per cent of your maximum heart rate. If you train too far below or above these figures, you will either not do much to condition your cardiovascular system or you will run the risk of injury. The THR can be estimated by subtracting your age from 220 and taking figures of 85 per cent and 70 per cent, respectively, from the resulting figure.

As with a car driver watching his rev counter, a runner should try to watch his heart rate to keep the needle around 90 per cent of his maximum heart rate to achieve cardiovascular conditioning and improvement with reduced risk of strain or subsequent illness. Another similarity with a car rev counter is that the needle will move according to the effort required to maintain a certain speed. Running uphill or running in humid conditions, for example, will raise the heartbeat, while the speed drops. Towards the end of a lengthy run, the heart rate will be raised due to fatigue and the subsequent strain placed on the heart, and ideally the training speed should be reduced to compensate. An efficient engine will be able to keep a certain speed with minimum revs per minute and a fit runner will also travel faster for the number of heartbeats per minute. Your can test your THR by feeling your pulse for 10 seconds after exercise and multiplying by six or by using a heart rate monitor.

Maximum Heart Rate

Maximum heart rate (MHR) is defined as the rate at which your heart can no longer satisfy increased demands for oxygen, or its maximum

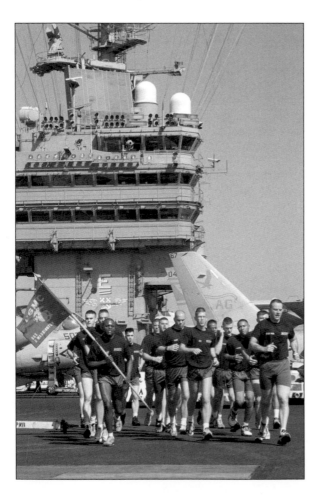

Left: Running is the basis of all fitness for military forces, and it is especially important for personnel – such as the US Marines seen here running on a carrier deck – to maintain their fitness for maximum readiness.

Brigade of Guards / Parachute Regiment Preparation Training Schedule

WEEK	MON	TUES	WED	THUR	FRI	SAT	SUN
1	• 20-minute run • Upper body exercises	Cycle/circuit training	• 40-minute run • Upper body exercises	Swimming/circuit training	• 20-minute run • Upper body exercises	Rest/easy/swim	Easy/swim
2	• 40-minute run • Upper body exercise	Cycle 60 minutes/circuit training	• 30-minute run • Upper body exercises	Circuit training/swim 60 minutes	• 2km (1¼-mile) = 15 minutes • 2km (1¼-mile) = best effort • Upper body exercises	Rest/easy swim	Easy/swim
3	• 2km (1¼-mile) = 15 minutes • 2km (1¼-mile) = best effort • Upper body exercises	Cycle 60 minutes/circuit training	• 40-minute run, steady • Upper body excrcises	Circuit training/swim 60 minutes	• 2km (1¼-mile) = 15 minutes • 2km (1¼-mile) = best effort • Upper body exercises	Rest/easy/swlɪɪ	Easy/swim
4	• 0.6km (1-mile) jog • 0.6km (1-mile) fast • 0.6km (1-mile) jog • 0.6km (1-mile) fast • Upper body exercises	Cycle 60 minutes/circuit training	• 40-minute run steady with hills • Upper body exercises	Circuit training/swim 60 minutes	• 0.6km (1-mile) jog • 0.6km (1-mile) fast • 0.6km (1-mile) jog • 0.6km (1-mile) fast • 5 x 100m sprints • Uppor body exercises	Rest/easy/swim	Easy/swim

beat rate. One way to estimate your MHR is by subtracting your age from 220. If you have a heart rate monitor, you can test your MHR by running hard for three minutes in two sessions, doing a pulse count after each run, with a relaxed jog between the sessions and after. This test should be done only if you are reasonably fit and thoroughly warmed up.

Frequency

If you are training as a runner and have reached a reasonable level of fitness which you wish to increase to attain your goals, then you should be running at least every other day, with serious runners running most days in succession with one day off each week. Should your goal be to join a military unit such as the Parachute Regiment or the US Marine Corps, these units prescribe preparation programmes that use running as the base activity and which also incorporate other training such as weights and swimming (see below). If these programmes are adhered to, you will arrive at the training unit much better able to cope with the programme and also far more liable to suffer less under the rigours of severe training.

Warming Up

Before you set out on your run, you should always go through a basic warm-up to condition and prepare your muscles. For many people, a few minutes of walking before a run is the best way to warm up. Warming up should be distinguished from stretching, which is a more elaborate process, Furthermore, many experts believe that stretching is best done after a run, rather than before.

Stretching

Stretching exercises reduce the tension in muscles, make them more flexible and improve the blood flow. If you are a runner, your stride will be increased and you will run more efficiently if

your leg muscles have be properly warmed up and stretched first.

A basic principle of stretching is not to bounce on the stretch. A taut muscle needs to be eased into a more flexible configuration, and this is best achieved by applying gentle and firm pressure to the point where the muscle begins to feel taut. (The point of pain is the indicator of how taut the muscle is.)

By holding the stretch for about 30 seconds at the taut stage, then repeating, you should gradually be able to push back the point of pain and deepen the stretch. When it comes to jumping a hurdle or leaping across a ditch on a cross-country run, the muscle should be flexible enough to cope, rather than cramping up with

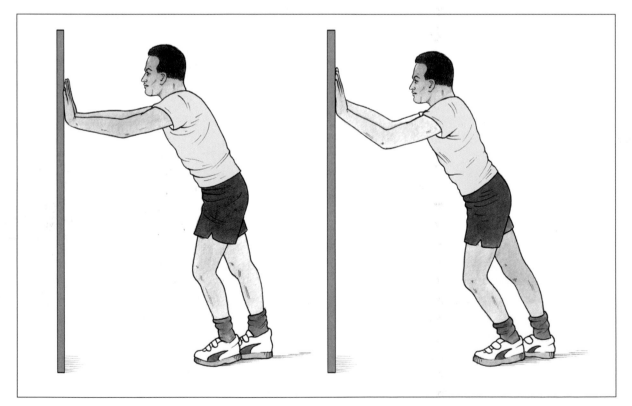

Above: To stretch your upper calves, stand about 1m (3ft) from a wall, placing your hands on the wall and feet flat on the ground. Bend your left knee and bring your heel off the ground. Keep your right knee straight and right foot flat on the ground. Lean forwards until you feel the stretch in your right calf. Repeat for left calf.

pain under the sudden strain. Stretching after a run has the benefit of providing a warm-down for muscles that may have become tight during the exercise.

It is said that time spent in planning is never wasted; the same can be said for stretching. Warmed-up and stretched muscles will work more efficiently and the athlete will be much less prone to injury. He or she is therefore likely to win against athletes who have taken shortcuts in this regard.

Stretching Exercises

1. Upper Calf: stand at least 1m (3ft) away from a wall and, keeping both feet flat on the ground, lean forward and place both palms of the hands on the wall, with your arms at right angles to the wall. Lift one heel off the ground by bending a knee while keeping the other leg straight and foot flat on the ground. Lean forward by bending your elbows until you feel the calf of your supporting leg stretch. Repeat the stretch with the other leg.

2. Lower Calf: stand close to a wall so that you can touch it without leaning forward. With one foot flat on the floor, bend the other leg. If you bend the other leg and lower the body, you will intensify the stretch.

3. Iliotibial band: standing sideways on to a wall; cross your legs to place one foot around the

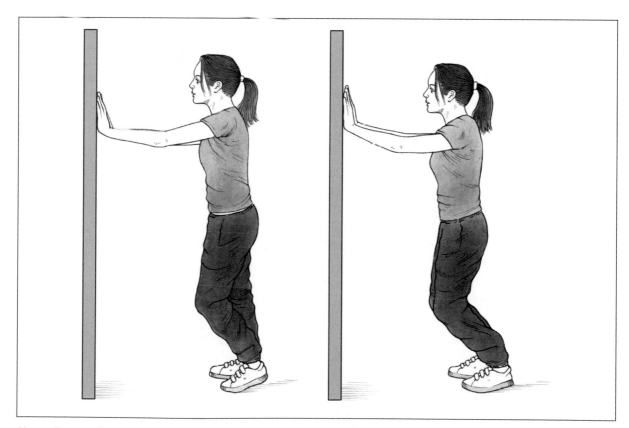

Above: For your lower calves, stand close to a wall and touch it with your palms. Bend the knee and lift the left heel.
Bend the right knee and lower your body till you feel the stretch near the bottom of the right calf. Repeat for left calf.

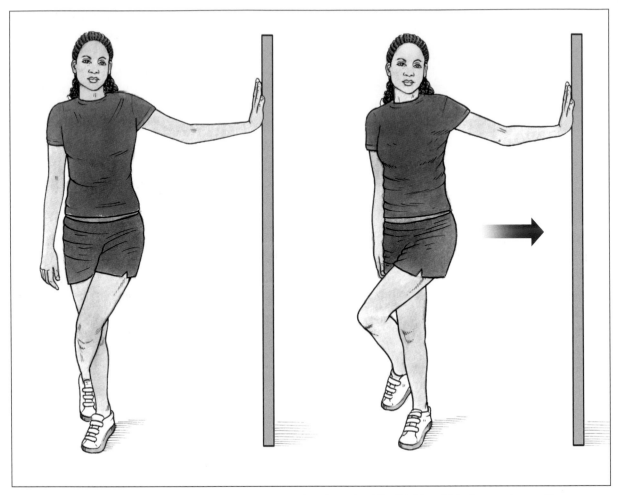

Above: The iliotibial stretch is an important one for reducing the risk of iliotibial band friction syndrome. Runners often suffer from this injury, which is also refered to as 'runner's knee'.

other. Lean towards the wall while supporting yourself with the palm of your right hand. With the right knee and elbow straight, push the hips towards the wall. You should feel a stretch down the side of the left thigh. Repeat the process for the other leg.

4. Shins: kneel with ankles and feet together. Gradually lower your body until you are sitting on your heels. Push your ankles down while keeping them together. You should feel the stretch in your shins.

5. Groin: sit on the ground and pull the soles of your feet together. Your hands should be on your feet and your elbows should be resting on your knees or thighs. Keeping a straight back, use your leg muscles to gradually force your knees towards the ground. You should feel a stretch in the groin. The effect is intensified the closer your feet are to your body.

6. Buttocks: lie on your back with your left leg straight. Bend your right leg until it comes back towards your hip. Rotate your right heel towards

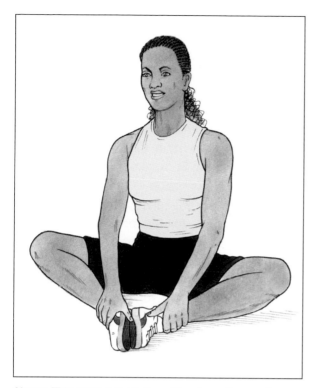

Above: This stretch is designed to strengthen and condition the gluteal muscles in the backside and improves their shape.

your left hip and hold your right ankle with your left hand and your right knee with your right hand. Pull the leg towards your shoulders until you feel the stretch in your right buttock. Repeat the process for your left buttock.

7. Hamstring: while lying on your back with one leg straight, bend the knee of your other leg and bring it back towards the hip. While the knee is still bent, grasp the hamstring of the raised leg and straighten the leg until you feel the stretch in your hamstring.

8. Thigh: lie on your stomach with one leg straight and the other bent at 90 degrees. Put a rope or towel round the raised ankle and hold with both hands. Push against the rope or towel

using the raised leg until you feel the stretch in your thigh. Repeat for the other thigh.

9. Standing quadriceps stretch: standing upright, bend one leg at the knee and catch your foot behind you. Flex your foot against your hands until you feel the stretch through the front of your leg.

11. Kneeling quadriceps stretch against a wall: with your back to a wall, pull one foot and shin up behind you and flatten them against the wall. Lean your body back to maximize the stretch.

13. Cross-legged sitting gluteal stretch: sit down on the ground and cross your legs, with your back straight. Pushing your feet out as far to the side as possible, bend forwards with arms outstretched.

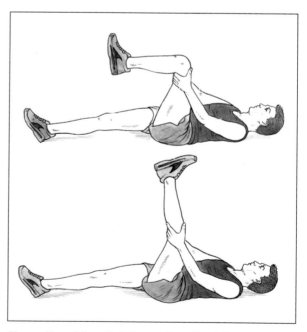

Above: Hamstring stretches reduce the risk of strains or pulls in these important muscles. It is vital to stretch the hamstring muscles before undertaking any exercise that involves running.

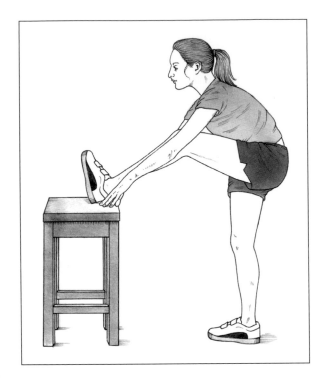

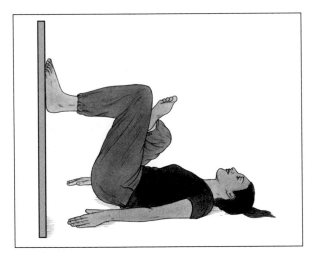

Above: Lying gluteal stretch against a wall – lie on your back with your buttocks about 1m (3ft) from a wall, allowing your lower back to be just off the ground. Place your feet against the wall, then cross one foot over to rest just below the knee of your other leg. As your body weight pulls towards the ground, you should feel a stretch in the muscles on the side of your buttocks.

Left: Bent-leg standing hamstring stretch – place one foot on a stable object such as a low wall. With a bent leg, bring your chest down towards your thigh, then gently attempt to straighten your bent leg.

Running

Few people would deny that running is the basis of most sports and that those who excel in a variety of sports, from tennis to rowing, use running as the foundation of their fitness. Some might argue that swimming provides an equally complete workout for the body, but it cannot be disputed that most sports are land-based and involve various forms of running or agility on the feet. In the military, every selection or recruit-training course uses running as the main element in building physical endurance. The training will involve early morning PT runs, running in boots within squads, running with or without assault vests and pouches, running with weights such as logs or stretchers, and running over obstacles such as assault courses, sometimes carrying a full load of equipment including a rifle and/or machine gun with all its requisite ammunition.

Ultimately, a soldier or a marine has to rely on his or her legs. This was demonstrated in the 1982 Falklands War where the conflict was not ultimately decided by sophisticated weaponry, but by infantry armed with rifles and bayonets. In one manoeuvre, British 45 Commando and 3 Para (3rd Battalion The Parachute Regiment) marched 64km (40 miles) in three days, each man carrying packs of up to 50kg (110lb). The terrain was difficult and at that time the British Army and Marines were equipped with a basic 'DMS' (Directly-Moulded Sole) ankle boot that provided little support, did not keep water out and had no cushioning properties.

The modern soldier has a much better deal, with calf-length boots made from supple water-

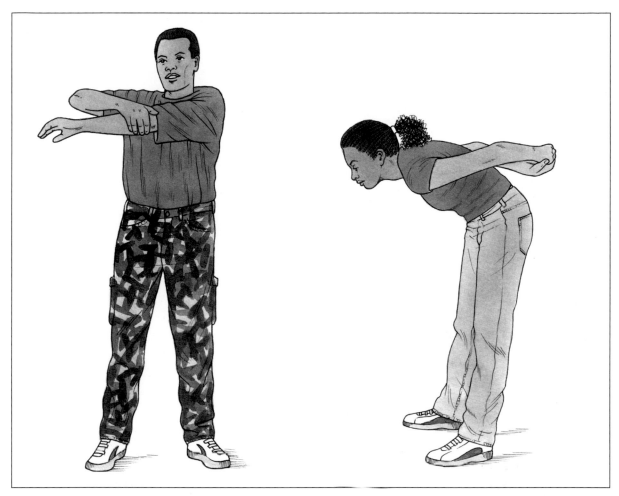

Above: It is important to stretch your anterior deltoid (shoulder) muscles before taking up any activity that involves use of the arms (left). To do this, graps the arm with your resting hand above the elbow and pull the arm into your chest, holding for 10 seconds. Repeat with the other arm. Stretching the pectoral (chest) muscles is also important (right). This can be achieved by fully extending your arms and clasping your hands behind your back, then leaning forward to stretch for about 10 seconds.

resistant leather and with mixed EVA and polyurethane soles developed from running-shoe technology. He can move much more quickly on his feet than his predecessors and with greatly reduced risk of foot infections or leg or back injuries. One factor, however, remains constant: the soldier standing in those boots needs to be fit enough to go the distance and every Physical Training Instructor (PTI) at Fort Bragg, Quantico, Lympstone, Pirbright or Hereford knows that the best way to achieve that fitness is by mile upon mile of running.

For training purposes, time spent running is more important than the distance covered, though the two are, of course, related. The important thing to remember is that you should neither overtrain nor undertrain. The body will adapt to gradually increased workloads and grow stronger,

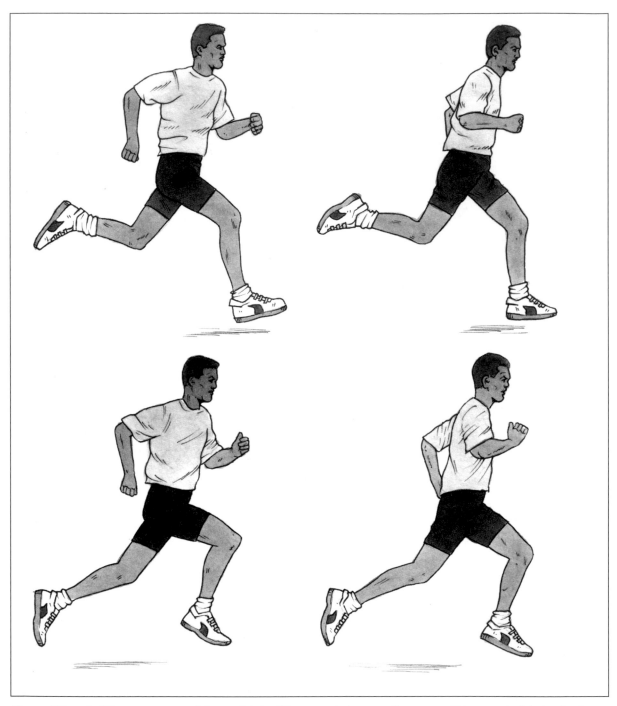

Above: Although different runners will have slightly different techniques, a fit person will have a straight back when running, with the legs going out in front of the body. The forearms should pump in a relaxed way at right angles to the ground. The rate of movement of your arms should mirror that of your legs. Breathe regularly; perhaps take some regulated breaths at the beginning of the run to gain control of your breathing before your start.

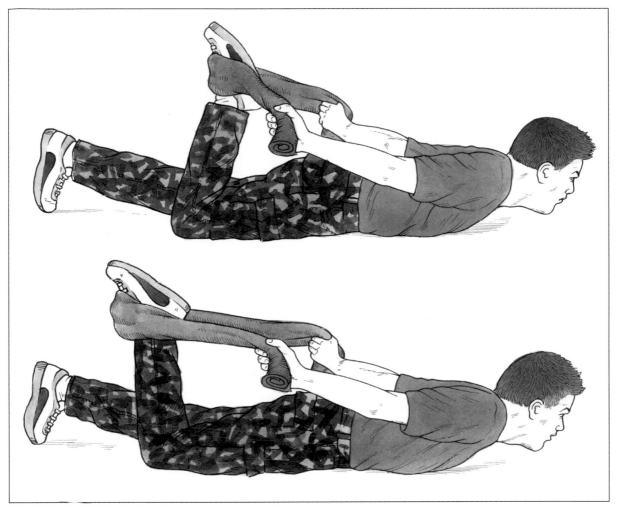

Above: Lying quad stretch – lying on your front, pull both arms back and place a towel or something similar round one foot. Push your foot against the towel until you feel the stretch in your quads.

but if it is forced to do too much too quickly it will quickly decline and the result will be fatigue and injury. Training must be both consistent and constant: you cannot expect to get to a certain level of fitness and stay there without further work. Your muscles will quickly re-adapt to a sedentary lifestyle if they are not given a regular workout.

There several different types of running training, each with its own accompanying benefits and disadvantages:

Long Runs

If you are training for a military selection programme, or for any endurance adventure, you will want to build a large number of long runs into your training schedule. Some people are well adapted to long runs and they are likely to fare well in the area of endurance; however, an endurance runner should also remember to utilize a fair measure of speed training in his schedules lest his body loses its ability to put on speed when required. Bear in mind that too much endurance training can have a negative effect by breaking down some muscle fibres. It is also thought that running a reasonable distance at a faster pace can have more benefit on your overall performance than running twice the distance at a slow rate. A wise practice is to introduce some faster-paced sessions within the context of the longer run. This alternation of speed allows your fast-twitch muscles to come into action and trains your body to produce speed when necessary. You can also divide up your run into separate sections with different speeds, so that your body experiences the full range of speedwork and endurance rather than concentrating on just one form of running.

Fartlek

Fartlek is derived from the Swedish word for 'speed play' and essentially it means adapting your speed in a more or less random way throughout the course of a run. Typically this may involve increasing your pace until you reach a certain tree or junction in a path or the other side of a field, then slowing down again until you feel ready for another burst of speed. The advantage of this kind of running is that it prepares the body for the unpredictable moments in a military training run or endurance race when you see an opportunity to get ahead of competitors. Essentially, you are training your body to change down from fifth gear to fourth or third and provide the extra accaleration and power when necessary.

Obviously, though, there are times when you feel like a tractor and do not feel inclined to try to behave like a sportscar, so another alternative to varying your pace and increasing your power is hill training.

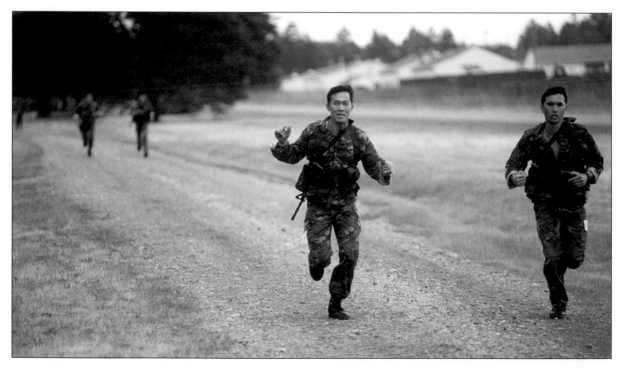

Above: Singapore army recruits take part in a 5km (3-mile) run. To prepare for military training programmes, it is important to familiarize yourself with running in boots and with equipment, such as belt kit and weapons.

Hill Training

Training on hills is an immensely beneficial way of increasing the training return on a measured distance. Hills are literally packed with fitness challenges, as they force your muscles to work harder to shift the commensurately greater load of your body against increased gravitational pull. It is a fact that hill training increases your muscles' ability to work hard for long periods. At risk of stating the obvious, hill training prepares you for running up hills, which have a particulary nasty habit of turning up repeatedly in any adventure. A good hill runner has an advantage over his opponents, as many people slow down on hills in much the same way as underpowered cars tend to do. Although these people may be able to run as quickly as most on the flat, hills will inevitably find them out, and show their lack of underlying power. If your muscles are trained for hill running, you will be able to use hills to get ahead of the pack, or to sustain your timeline despite the added challenge they represent.

Resistance Training

This form of training has a similar effect to hill training in that it increases the load on your muscles. For military recruits this form of training makes sense, as it mimics the kind of loads that will be experienced when carrying a bergen or pack, assault vests, weapons and ammunition. If the body is used to carrying a greater weight in training, it should be better prepared to cope with actual challenges.

As with long-distance running, however, there is a word of caution to be noted here. Too much work with weights can instil a slow, plodding style of running that will be detrimental to performance in timed sessions requiring speed as well as endurance. Resistance training, therefore, should be used as part of a variety of training resources.

United States Navy SEALs Suggested Running Training Schedule I

WEEK	
1	3km (2 miles) per day (Mon, Wed, Fri) = 10km (6 miles) per week
2	Ditto
3	No running
4	5km (3 miles) per day (Mon, Wed, Fri) = 14km (9 miles) per week
5	Mon: 3km (2 miles) Tues: 5km (3 miles) Thurs: 6km (4 miles) Fri: 3km (2 miles) Total: 17km (11 miles)
6	Ditto
7	Mon: 6km (4 miles) Tues: 6km (4 miles) Thurs: 8km (5 miles) Fri: 5km (3 miles) Total: 25km (16 miles)
8	Ditto
9	Ditto

Striding

This form of running is fast and economical, once you get into your stride, if you will forgive the pun. When striding, you are essentially in fifth gear, cruising at a good speed on the flat. The aim is to train your legs to accept a high rate of running, and therefore striding is the opposite of the 'plodding' of a long-distance run. Depending on your fitness, you can stride for anything between 100 and 400m (328 and 1312ft), then jog to recover.

Stride training will pay off big dividends when you are in the optimum position in a race, the time when perhaps you have done most of the hard work necessary, but what you need to do at that point is to turn on the speed in a final sprint for home and a hot shower.

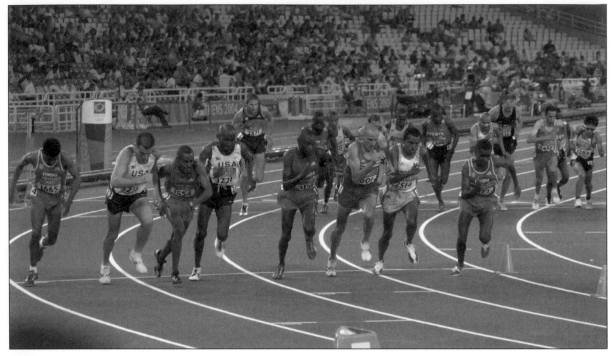

Above: Captain Dan Browne of the US Oregon National Guard (second left) at the start of the 10,000m final of the 2004 Athens Olympics. The high levels of fitness demanded by military forces can produce star athletes.

Speed Training

Those who are intending to join the armed forces will not necessarily need to concentrate on speed training. The military demands endurance over long distance and values the ability to do a job of work at the end of it. The advantage of speed or sprint training, however, is that it can contribute to the development of the body musculature and enable you to put on a turn of speed when necessary.

The three main competitive speed events – 100, 200 and 400 metres – each require their own special skills, but there is no harm in building them into your schedule if you want to add another string to your bow.

Note that if you are unable to access natural land on which to run, a good gym will usually have treadmill facilities. Even marathon runners use treadmills for both endurance training and speedwork. There are many elements of land running that are missing on a treadmill, but it can be used successfully either for precise tuning or for interval training.

Cross Training

Although running has numerous advantages, it also has some limitations. Due to the fact that the body is totally unsupported, fatigue can set in comparatively quickly during intensive training and the need to take a rest interval can limit your overall aerobic training. In addition, although running is a complete sport that provides an excellent fitness foundation, it does not develop all of the muscles of the body equally, particularly those in the upper body. Running, therefore, should be mixed with other sporting activities. Different sports tend to focus on different muscle groups, so cross training is very useful in increasing overall performance and preventing injuries in a base sport such as running. Sports such as biking and langlauf (cross-country skiing), for example, will help to develop the quadriceps muscles, while swimming can strengthen the lower back and rowing and race-walking develop the abdominal muscles.

Swimming

Swimming competes with running for all-round muscle conditioning. The advantage swimming has over running is that the water provides support for the body and therefore the kind of impact injuries commonly experienced by runners are not an issue. The recovery rate from swimming exercise is also much quicker than from running. Indeed, swimming is used extensively as a means of working up muscle strength after injuries experienced in other activities. Swimming can therefore be inserted into the training schedule as an alternative to running and also to allow the body to recover from its running schedule. It cannot, however, be used to replace running entirely, as there are certain muscle groups that can only be strengthened by a running regime.

Swimming is technically more complex than running, with numerous different stroke techniques. Although handbooks will enable you to understand the dynamics of the strokes, it is advisable to seek the help of a coach if you are not experienced. For the purposes of training and fitness, a good command of breaststroke and front crawl will suffice, the latter being technically more difficult than the former due to the need for correct breathing technique.

As with running, it is a good idea to do at least a minimum amount of warming up, including some stretching, before you get in the pool. Once in the water, you can continue the warm-up by having a gentle swim to get the muscles

working properly. Your workout may involve sets of lengths with five to 10 seconds in between, depending on your level of fitness. A major set should be followed by a warm-down swim of about 100m (328ft).

For those at base level of fitness, you should be aiming to swim between four and five days per week and covering about 200m (656ft) per session. This can be broken down as:

Week 1	15 minutes' continuous swimming
Week 2	15 minutes' continuous swimming
Week 3	20 minutes' continuous swimming
Week 4	20 minutes' continuous swimming
Week 5	25 minutes' continuous swimming
Week 6	25 minutes' continuous swimming
Week 7	30 minutes' continuous swimming
Week 8	30 minutes' continuous swimming
Week 9	35 minutes' continuous swimming

For those at a more advanced level of fitness, or who have graduated from the base-level programme, the next series might look like this:

Week 1	35 minutes' continuous swimming
Week 2	35 minutes' continuous swimming
Week 3	45 minutes' continuous swimming
Week 4	45 minutes' continuous swimming
Week 5	60 minutes' continuous swimming
Week 6	75 minutes' continuous swimming

If you are an experienced swimmer, you will already know enough about swimming workouts to build from there. Effectively there are as many swimming workouts as there are swimmers, and everyone will eventually work out their favourite techniques or pick their favourite workouts devised by coaches or found in specialist books. The following workouts are based on a standard Olympic dimensions swimming pool – 25 x 50m (82 x 164ft).

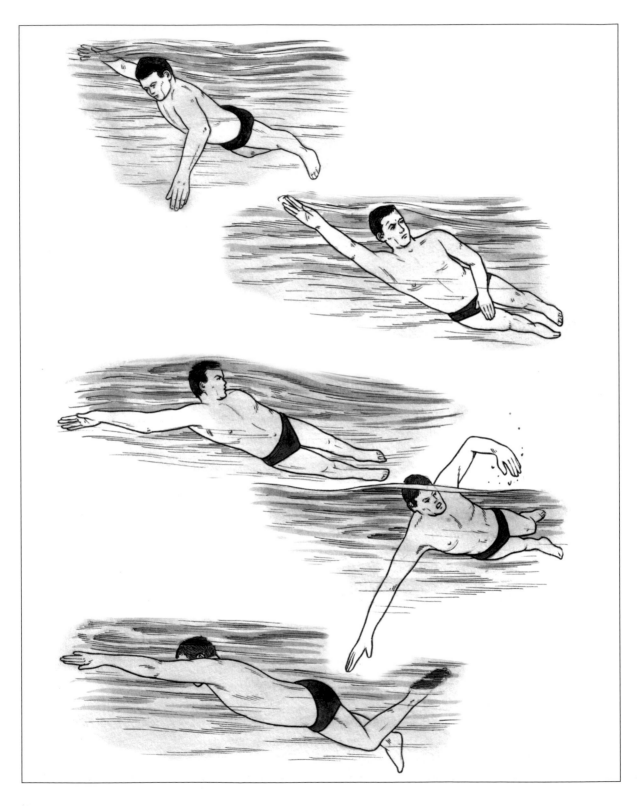

Front Crawl

The front crawl is the fastest swimming stroke, and if you are thinking of competing in something like a triathlon you will need to get to grips with it sooner rather than later, as it will pay dividends in the biking and running sessions. The energy saved from having an efficient stroke and good technique will pay huge dividends.

Unlike running, where wind resistance is not a major factor (you can do very little about it in any case), swimming has a great deal to do with minimizing water resistance on the body. The best way to do this is to keep your body as flat as possible in the water, which helps to reduce drag. You should keep your head as steady as possible, letting it turn with the rest of your body when you come up for breath.

In essence, the crawl involves pushing one arm straight out in front of you in the water, like the prow of a ship, and using the other to push your body forward. You should exert a strong, consistent stroke with the arm in the water, bending your elbow slightly as you feel the pressure of the water against your hand and pulling it firmly outwards, inwards and backwards, taking an S-shape line towards your thigh. When the arm has gone through the full stroke and is coming out of the water, brushing your thigh as it exits, the arm that has been the prow is already pushing down for another stroke. At this point the body may be at an angle of 45 degrees as the swimmer lifts one arm out of the water and takes a breath of air. The body then

Opposite: When performing front crawl or freestyle, keep your body as close to the surface as possible; bend your knees slightly and kick long and fast; stretch one arm straight out in front and cut it cleanly into the water; bend your elbow and push your hand towards your feet; brush the side of your thigh with your hand as you bring it out of the water at the end of the stroke.

United States Navy SEALs Suggested Swimming Schedule I

WEEK	
1	15 minutes' continuous swimming
2	15 minutes' continuous swimming
3	20 minutes' continuous swimming
4	20 minutes' continuous swimming
5	25 minutes' continuous swimming
6	25 minutes' continuous swimming
7	30 minutes' continuous swimming
8	30 minutes' continuous swimming
9	35 minutes' continuous swimming

rolls towards the lifted arm, which is pushed out in front. The body roll should be a natural action involving the whole body and caused by the pressure of the arm reaching into the water below your chest and pulling back. When you recover your hand from the water, your elbow should emerge first, pointing up towards the sky. As your hand moves forwards again to the front of your body, your fingers should brush the surface of the water.

Although the front crawl is, as the name suggests, mostly about arms, your legs perform an absolutely vital role, and if the leg movement is incorrect the whole balance of the stroke is upset. You will exert the greatest force with your legs if you think in terms of moving the whole leg from the hip downwards, rather than focusing on your feet and the bottom of your legs, although it is easy to do this because it is at the bottom of the legs that you most feel the impact of the water. Your thighs are the heaviest and widest part of your leg, and if you are moving them efficiently you will be exerting considerable supportive power. Your knees should be slightly bent, in order to keep your leg flexible. The speed of your legs in the water will dictate the speed of your arms, so do not try small fast kicks with your legs when you want to do slow powerful sweeps with your arms. Fast kicks are for those moments when you need to sprint. Your legs throughout should be close together, which aids streamlining through the water.

Different swimmers have different methods of breathing: some will breathe on every stroke, while others will take a breath after every two or every four strokes. Some swimmers breathe on

Sample Workouts

Workout A	
Dry Warm-up	Concentrating on your biceps, triceps and pectorals, and including a stretch of the back muscles
Pool Warm-up	200m split as 50m freestyle, 50 m breaststroke, 50m freestyle, 50m breaststroke
Preamble to the Main Set	100m with a frog-kick; 100m breaststroke drill; 100m breaststroke swim
Main Set	4 x 50m breaststroke sprints
Warm-down	150m freestyle

Workout B	
Warm-up: Freestyle	4 x 200m with each 200m lap being incrementally faster than the last one, for example Lap Two 2.5 seconds faster than Lap One; Lap Three 3.5 seconds faster than Lap Two; Lap Four 4.5 seconds faster than Lap Three
Butterfly	200m, focusing on the kick (front, back and side); 100m butterfly with the right arm; 100m butterfly with the left arm; swim 2 x 50m with normal stroke
Backstroke	100m with delayed pull, focusing on kick on side; swim 100m with normal stroke
Breaststroke	100m normal stroke; 100m with a dolphin kick
Freestyle	4 x 75m focusing on pull; 200 yards focusing on kick
Warm-down	100m

Workout C	
Freestyle	3 x 100m with 25 second rests 3 x 75m with 20 second rests 3 x 50m with 15 second rests 3 x 25m with 10 second rests
Multiple	Free, fly, free: 7: Free, back, free Free, breaststro Fly, backstroke,
Breaststroke	Pull: 150m Drills: 150m Normal stroke: 6 x 50m
Freestyle	Kick: 6 x 25m Pull: 100m focusing on number of strokes (i.e. fewer strokes per set distance)
Warm-down	100m

just one side of the body, while others breathe on both sides. The argument in favour of the latter is that it will tend to make your movement through the water more even. For each breath you take you should rotate your body in the water at an angle of no more than 45 degrees. To exhale the air you have already taken in, wait until you are at least halfway through the stroke and your head is turning towards the side on its way up to the surface. Once your head is clear of the surface of the water you can exhale the remaining air and clear your nose and mouth. If the timing is correct, your arm will have created a furrow in the water parallel to your body, and this can create extra space for you to breathe in a fresh lungful of air without having to exaggerate the movement of the head. When the arm that is out of the water comes forward, it should extend straight in front of your body, and the body should roll over onto that side.

Breaststroke

The breaststroke is much easier to perform than front crawl/freestyle, mostly because the breathing involved is far more straightforward, as the head is coming well clear of the water, allowing plenty of time to take a good breath. In breaststroke all the limbs work in unison, the arms and legs performing exactly the same movement in a synchronized fashion. Some people, however, may find this aspect of breastroke more difficult than the mixed arm and leg movements of front crawl/freestyle.

As with front crawl, you need to try to keep your body as level as possible and as close to the surface as possible in order to reduce drag. The shoulders and hips should be in line and flat. The leg movement is effectively the same as that of a frog. The legs kick outwards with the feet flat against the water, go round in a circular motion, then come back together again at the

United States Navy SEALs Suggested Sidestroke Swimming Schedule I

WEEK	
1	15 minutes' continuous swimming
2	15 minutes' continuous swimming
3	20 minutes' continuous swimming
4	20 minutes' continuous swimming
5	25 minutes' continuous swimming
6	25 minutes' continuous swimming
7	30 minutes' continuous swimming
8	30 minutes' continuous swimming
9	35 minutes' continuous swimming

end of the motion. At this point the legs should be straight and the knees touching each other. The arm movement begins with the arms stretched out in front. They are then swept outwards and round in a circle that is always drawn in front of the shoulders. Both arms are then pushed forwards again for the next stroke, known as the stretch. As you stretch, your face should be in the water, as this helps to keep the body flat and near the surface.

Breaststroke is all about maximizing power in each stroke, and it is not a stroke that should be performed hurriedly. To gain more speed in the breaststroke you need to increase the power of each stroke and the efficiency of movement of the body, and this can be helped by undulating. When you pull back with your arms, your head and shoulders clear the water and you then dive forwards. This creates an undulating movement, not dissimilar to the movement of a dolphin through water, which aids the forward movement. After bringing your hands together following a smooth and powerful sweep, keep your elbows

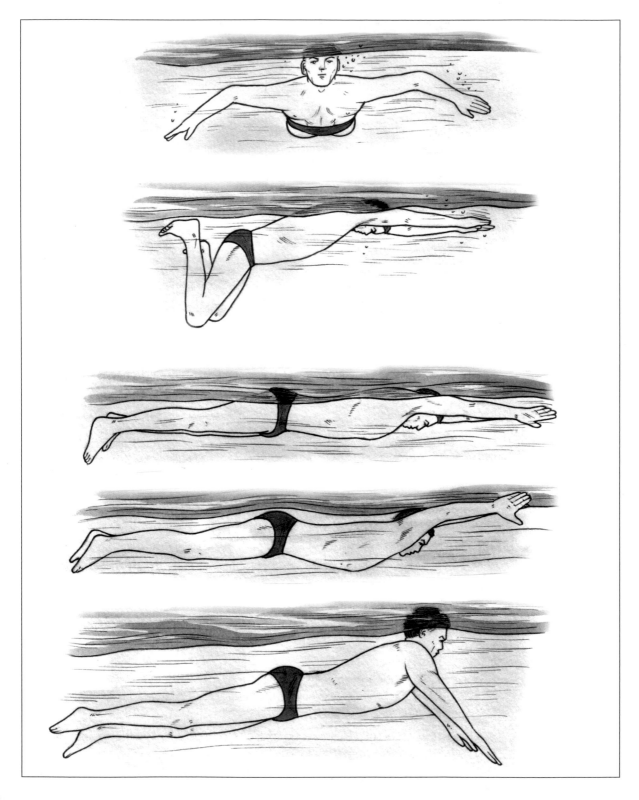

into your chest, to enhance streamlining. Your legs should go outside your body when you kick, but not so far that they create a counter-thrust against forward momentum.

Sidestroke

The sidestroke is taught particularly to those involved with maritime elite forces, as it is a useful stroke for use while pulling objects or other people in the water. For the sidestroke you can lie on either your left or your right side. During forward movement, the head, back and legs are kept straight, with the toes pointed, and the bottom arm is extended parallel with the surface of the water, palm of the hand facing down. The other arm is extended down over the top thigh. Your nose and mouth should be just clear of the water.

Both arms work alternately in the sidestroke and in different ways. The top arm is brought back along the body until it is in front of your top shoulder. The hand is then pushed downwards slightly and then back, until it is fully extended for the glide. The hand on the bottom arm should be pointed downwards and outwards. Bend the elbow and sweep the hand slightly downwards. The hand should come down under the bottom ear. Then slide the hand and arm back out in front of you, for the glide position.

The leg action in the sidestroke is fairly easy if you remember that each leg does precisely the

Opposite: For the breaststroke, keep your body level and as close to the surface as possible; pull your feet up to your bottom and push your feet out and inwards, with the flat of the feet against the water; straighten your legs with knees together for the glide; stretch arms out in front; draw a full circle with your hands, always keeping them in sight in front of your shoulders; and remember to keep limbs under the water and bring your head up to breathe.

COMBAT SIDESTROKE

The combat sidestroke is faster than normal sidestroke and is based on the stroke used by elite forces. This form of the sidestroke also allows good visibility and controlled breathing when swimming in rough seas. The main difference is that the swimmer rotates his head to the side and inhales while recovering the top arm, then replaces his head in the water while pushing back with the top arm and kicking backwards with the legs. In this way, the breathing cycle is similar to that used in freestyle.

opposite of the other. While the top leg kicks forwards, the bottom leg kicks back. Both of your knees are flexed as the feet go forwards and backwards. Power is delivered against the water by the sole of the top foot and by the top of the bottom foot. Once the leg and foot movement is complete, both toes should be pointed for the glide.

You should breathe in while you are recovering your limbs from each stroke, and exhale during the power push. If you are swimming with military or naval equipment in operations, you will need to follow your specific training, which may include swimming with your head pointed directly upwards.

Cycling

Cycling makes an excellent alternative to running. Part of the reason for this is that it exercises the muscles you would normally use in running, as well as others, in a supported way; the bike, after all, is taking the strain of the weight of your body, leaving you free to give your muscles a workout. Before riding, you should remember to warm up properly, as you would for any other exercise.

You can devise your own training programme, perhaps on the lines of five minutes at 10km (6 miles) pace, or even more intense shorter sessions of one minute at 5km (3 miles) pace, with a 30-second break in between each effort. You can increase the intervals as you grow fitter. Enthusiastic cyclists use running, weights and swimming as part of their fitness training, so the benefits are interchangeable. As with running, cycling offers a range of training possibilities according to distance and terrain, and you can place different levels of stress on your body according to your use of the gears.

Adjusting the Cycle

Cycling can serve up some novel injuries for the novice, as well as for experienced riders. Although the body is supported on the bike, if the bike is not set up in the optimum configuration for your size, you may end up with a positional injury.

One obvious source of discomfort is the saddle. A well-padded gel saddle which is wide enough to support your body should solve the problem. Because the cyclist is leaning forwards on his or her hands, problems may also arise in the nerves of the fingers. Avoid such injuries by adjusting the saddle height to reduce the amount of body weight supported by the hands, and regularly change the position of your hands on the handlebars – this will allow the blood to flow and reduce the pressure on the nerve at any particular point. Neck and back pains can result from poor positioning on the bike, as well as from the failure to stretch and warm up effectively before you start.

Runners who suffer from knee pain may be disappointed to find that they can pick up similar injuries on a bike. Again, this may be due to lack of proper stretching and warm-up. Another cause may be that your saddle may be too low, thus forcing your knees to take too much of the pressure. To minimize the chance of injury and discomfort, and to maximize your cycling efficiency, it is important to have the right size of bike (this normally means the correct frame size) and to adjust the seat and handlebars in such a way as to optimize your leg push and recovery.

If you sit on the bike with both feet on the pedals, supporting yourself against something steady, you can turn the pedal to its lowest point and place your heel on it. At this point your leg should be almost straight, with only a slight bend at the knee. If the knee is completely locked it means that the saddle is too high; conversely, if your knee is too bent it means the saddle is too low.

Ideally, the saddle should be parallel to the ground. This will prevent you from tipping and sliding either forwards or backwards. You can also test whether your saddle needs adjusting forwards or backwards by bringing the pedal round until it is at a three-o'clock position. There should now be a direct line down from your knee to the ball of your foot. If this is not the case, adjust the saddle either way. This is not an absolute rule, however, as your saddle position will determine the level of your crouch over the handlebars, which has obvious aerodynamic implications. It also has an impact on the way you use your gluteus maximus muscles. The further back your saddle is positioned, the more horizontal will be your body position. The saddle position should be such that you will achieve

Opposite: Cycling is good resistance training for runners as well as a sport in its own right. It can help you to develop powerful leg muscles, as well as provide an excellent workout for the heart and lungs.

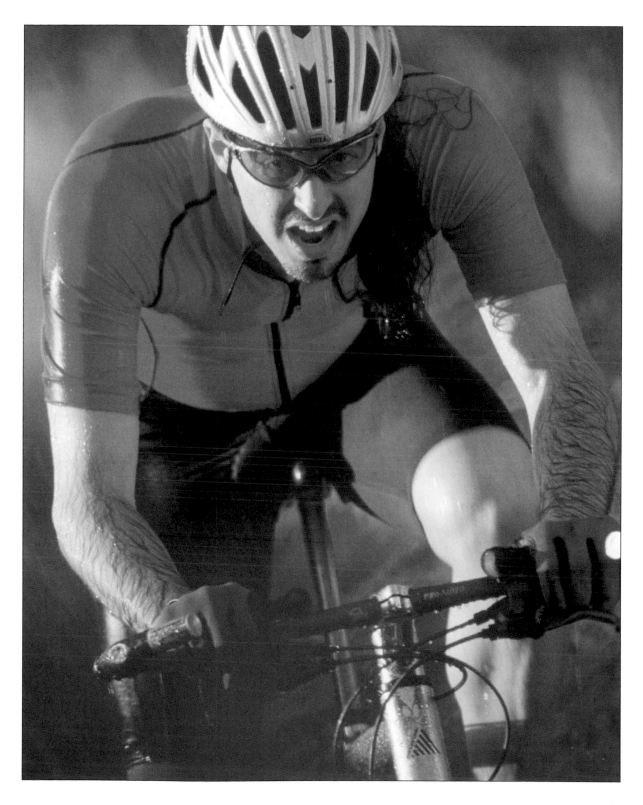

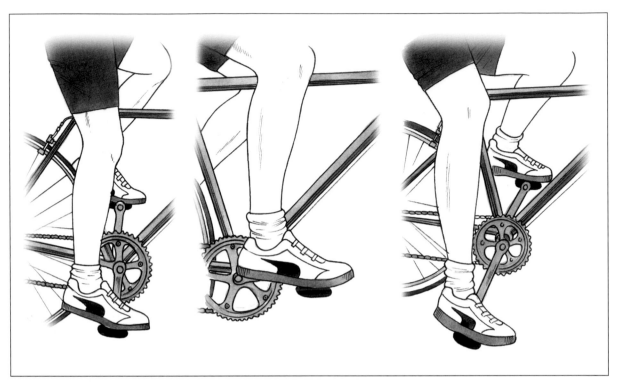

Above: Correct adjustment of the saddle is vital in cycling. Ideally, the knee should be slightly bent when the foot is on the pedal at the bottom of the stroke.

the optimum aerodynamic position, and the optimum amount of power into the pedals without having to lean too heavily on your arms and thus cause fatigue.

To adjust the handlebars, place your elbow against the front end of the saddle and point your arm towards the handlebars, then place your other hand across your fingertips at 90 degrees. The outside of the little finger on the hand at 90 degrees is approximately the position your handlebars should be at.

Again, the position of the handlebars is determined by your intended use of the bike. If the handlebars are farther forward, you will have more power if you have to stand up to pedal uphill. If the handlebars are set low, you will have a better aerodynamic position and you will be able to pull hard for good acceleration. The closer

the handlebars are to the seat and the higher they are, the more upright your position will be. As a general rule, touring bikers have their handlebars set about level with the saddle, while racing bikers tend to have them set at 5–7.6cm (2–3in) below the saddle. Mountain bikers generally have the bars about 5cm (2in) below the saddle.

Rowing

Rowing is an excellent way of improving strength and mobility, as well as cardiovascular efficiency. If you do not happen to have access to a pair of sculls and a river, you can opt for a rowing machine, either at your local gymnasium or by investing in one to have at home.

Rowing has the majority of its effort focused in the legs (about 70 per cent) and a significant though reduced amount in the upper body (about 30 per cent). For the rowing to be an efficient and beneficial exercise, this balance should be maintained. You should always go through the normal warm-up and stretching regimes before sitting down to a session on a rowing machine. As with any other sport, this prepares the muscles for the exercise and helps them to perform more efficiently.

When you start on the rowing machine, your forearms should be more or less parallel with the ground and the 'oar' or handle pulled in towards your midriff. Your legs should be fully stretched and you should be leaning back slightly. At the next stage, let your body move forwards, rotating from the hips, with the arms fully extended. This is the easy part, where in a boat the oars or sculls would be above the water. Next you should follow up this movement by bringing the rest of your body forward on the sliding seat.

When you are fully forward, your knees and upper legs should be against your chest and your lower legs should be at 90 degrees from the floor. Your arms remain straight. At this point you start to push with your legs while your upper body also pulls back from the hips to enhance the pull. Remember, it is the legs that are responsible for delivering most of the power. Still keeping most of the strain on your legs, continue to pull back with your upper body, keeping your arms straight at all times. Only when your legs are fully stretched and your upper body is leaning back do your bend your arms and pull the rowing handle in towards your midriff again. You should then be in the position you started. The next and consecutive strokes follow on from there.

There are, of course, differences between rowing on an indoor rowing machine and rowing on the water. Obviously, open-boat rowing involves lifting oars out of the water, which entails a different style of arm movement, with the elbows tending to splay outwards. You can

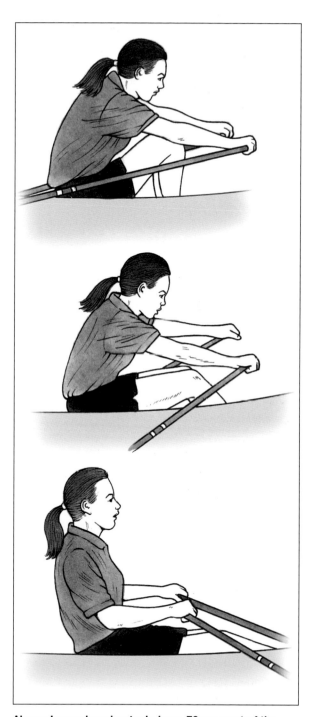

Above: In good rowing technique, 70 per cent of the power in rowing comes from the legs. Keep your arms straight until leaning slightly back, then bend the arms to pull the oars into your midriff.

adapt your technique quite easily with practise. In rowing, as with swimming, the technique is almost wholly responsible for the efficiency of the exercise (if it is a rowing machine) or to the movement of the boat (if you are on the water).

When rowing in a boat, the greater propulsive power is achieved when you lift the oars from the water and your body weight is driving towards the direction of movement. When you travel back towards your foot plate for recovery, a force is exerted in the opposite direction, against the forward momentum of the boat. One way of reducing the negative force on the boat – in other words, reducing the jarring body

TRIATHLON

Mixing some of the training elements mentioned above, namely running, swimming and cycling, can make you a likely contender for the triathlon. Triathlon is a growth sport that attracts athletes of all ages. There are a variety of reasons for the interest in this sport: one may stem purely from the fact that, as I have recommended in this book, athletes simply want to try a more stimulating mix of competition sport rather than focusing exclusively on one discipline. Triathlon gives you the opportunity to find a competitive dimension for that mixed fitness training.

The first test of your commitment as a triathlete will probably be financial. Unfortunately, triathlon bikes are specialized and therefore expensive. Some triathlon bikes use what are known as tri-bars, or aero bars, which allow the rider to lean forwards on the handlebars, with the backs of the elbows almost touching the knees. This position is similar to that adopted by downhill skiiers and it has the advantage of reducing the amount of your frontal area exposed to the wind, thus improving your overall aerodynamics by reducing drag. Triathlon bikes tend also to be configured with a comparatively high saddle position. With the body leaning forwards and the rear end high in the saddle, optimum power is smoothly transferred through the pedals.

Depending on how committed you are, you can set up similar angles on a traditional bike frame – a practical step if you are just using triathlon as part of your training programme and not necessarily making a long-term competitive investment. There are bits that can be added to a conventional bike, such as three-spoke wheels and tri-bars, that will help it to pass muster as a professional triathlon bike. Note that the swimming part of the triathlon will also require a certain amount of financial investment, including a racing swimsuit, a thin wetsuit for cold climes and anti-mist goggles.

Training for a triathlon obviously means training in all three disciplines, but they do not necessarily all require the same amount of time commitment. If you are already a fairly proficient runner, you will probably need to invest more time in such aspects as accustoming yourself to the rig of a triathlon bike and getting your cycling muscles warmed up and conditioned. As mentioned earlier, poor technique in swimming can have a disproportionate effect on your performance, so you may need to spend some time and money on getting your front crawl sorted out, in particular the movement of the body through the water and the breathing technique. You cannot just wing it with the crawl, particularly if you are swimming in the open sea, as poor technique will soon find you out.

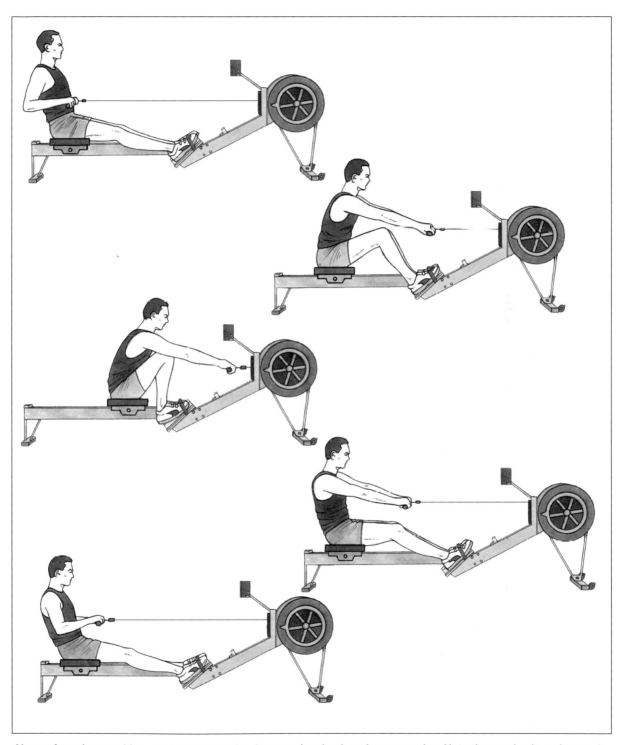

Above: A rowing machine can help you to develop your leg, back and arm muscles. Note the emphasis on leg work – the arms only bend at the end of the pull.

movement against the boat's direction of travel during the recovery stroke – is to distribute some of that force on to the oar blades that are re-entering the water. Some of the negative effect can therefore be neutralized by positive action with the oars. As sculling and rowing techniques are complex, they must be learned through coaching and plenty of practice.

Weight Training

Weight training is an important part of the preparation for military training programmes, and it also works for athletes across a variety of sports, including running, swimming and rowing. As most people lead relatively sedentary lives in urban environments, their muscles adapt to the moderate level of physical resistance that they encounter on a daily basis. Pushing pens or tapping keyboards does not build muscle.

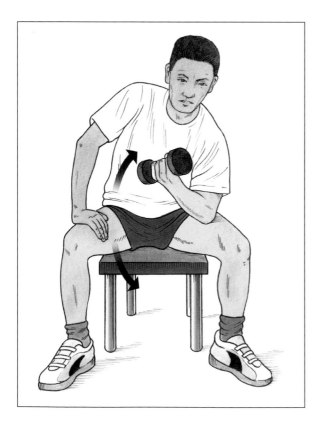

Weight training essentially replaces the kind of resistance work that might be encountered by someone working on a farm or building site, where lifting weights or pushing heavy loads is part of the daily routine.

Weights build up muscle and increase power. Soldiers need to be able to carry weights of up to 40kg (90lb) on their backs, in addition to the weight of their weapons, and they also need to be able to dig trenches and negotiate obstacles such as those found on assault courses. A well-developed upper body may mean the difference between hanging onto the monkey bars or falling in the cold water. Weight training will also make a difference to running speed, as an upper body that is well conditioned will work more efficiently with a running action and help to improve overall performance. There is a direct relationship between the swing of the arms and the movement of the legs. Although different runners tend to have different running styles, especially with regard to their arms, there is no doubt that, when going for the finish line, powerful arm movements provided by a strong upper body will make a considerable difference to your performance. A well-developed upper body will also help you to achieve better balance when running over uneven ground. Good leg muscles act like shock absorbers and reduce the risk of injury when you are running on uneven ground or downhill.

Correct running posture depends on the upper body being kept more or less erect, while the legs get on with the running. Strong stomach muscles and other abdominal muscles help to maintain optimum posture. Those who suffer

Left: For concentration curls, sit on a bench with one barbell in one hand. Place your elbow on your leg and pull the barbell towards your shoulder, before lowering again. Repeat at least 10 times on each side.

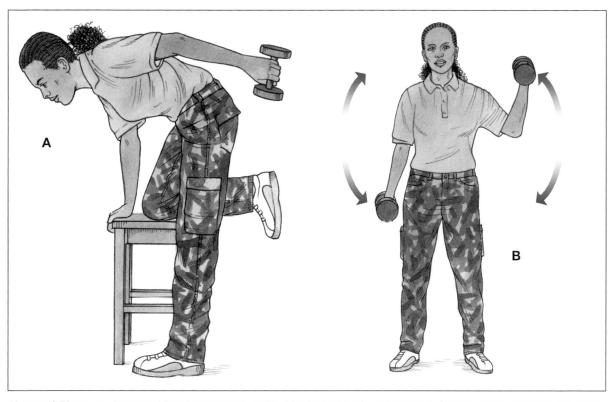

Above: A) Place one knee and hand on a stool, and hold a barbell in the other hand. Starting with your arm hanging straight towards the ground, raise it backwards to shoulder level. Bring it back to the straight-down position and repeat. B) Hold both barbells by your side, and alternately raise each arm to bring the barbell up to chest height.

from back injuries often look in the wrong place – the back – for the source of the problem. The cause of the back ache is often to be found in the region of the stomach and abdomen, where inadequately developed muscles have failed to support the back properly, leading to overstrain on the muscles of the back and the spine. Weight training can correct this problem, and have a positive effect on your bones as well, partly because better developed muscles support the bone structure and partly because the healthy pull of muscle on bone tends to help bones to regenerate. A well-conditioned and strong body is a body that suffers less strain due to the fact that it can cope with more for less effort. This in turn means less strain on the heart.

A word of caution should be made here: if you are unfit or have any form of heart condition, treat weights with extreme caution and seek advice from a medical practitioner and coach before taking on a weight-training programme. Furthermore, weight training should not be confused with body building. Weight training is based on frequent repetitions of relatively modest weights, while body building is concerned with short, sharp bursts with very heavy weights. Weight training is about the conditioning and development of muscles throughout the body in order to optimize the performance in a range of activities. The end view in strength training is to increase the strength of your muscles; this is accompanied by an expansion in muscle mass.

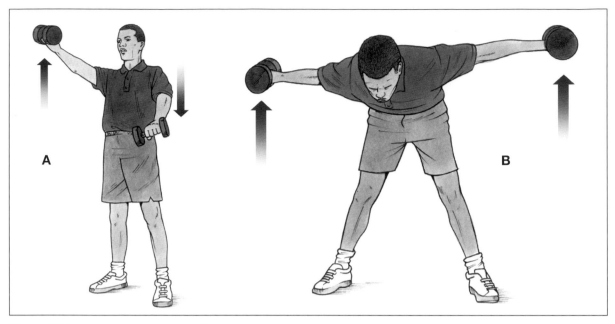

Above: A) Hold the barbells by your side. Alternately raise and lower your arms from the side to the horizontal position. Keep the body straight. B) Bend forwards, keeping your back straight. Holding the barbells, raise both arms to the horizontal, then lower them. Keep the top part of your body completely straight and the knees slightly

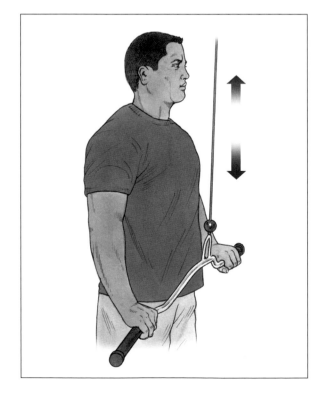

Through weight training endurance of your muscles is increased by improvements in the blood flow to the muscles.

The repetitions that are performed with weights will improve the strength and endurance of a particular muscle group. You then move on to another piece of equipment, or use your dumb bells in a different way in order to work on and develop a different muscle group. In general, sets should be repeated at least three times per session for the maximum benefit. As with running and other exercises, it is a good thing to build in a rest period, allowing time for the muscle tissue to build up after the breaking down of the exercise session.

Left: To perform press-downs, hold the bar with both hands and press it down with a smooth motion, using only your arm muscles. Let the bar rise again in a controlled manner, and repeat.

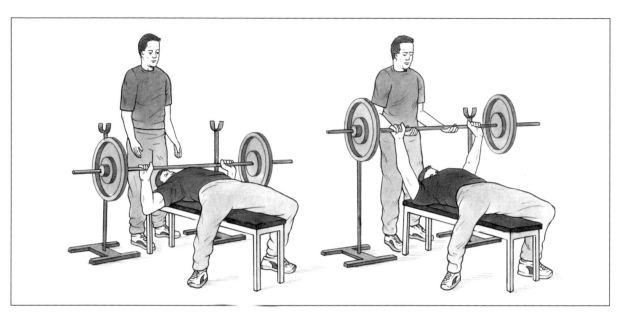

Above: To perform a bench press, lie on your back with your shoulders directly under the weight. Keep your back flat. Raise the weights until your arms are straight. If it is a free weight, have a trainer on stand-by to help. Repeat.

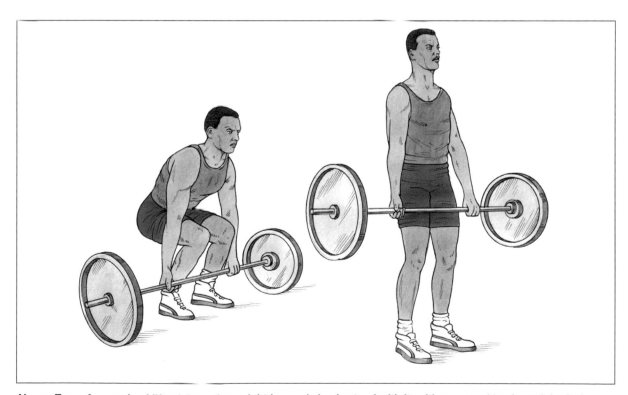

Above: To perform a dead lift, pick up the weight bar and simply stand with it, with arms and back straight, before replacing it on the ground in a controlled manner. This exercise will strengthen your back and quadriceps.

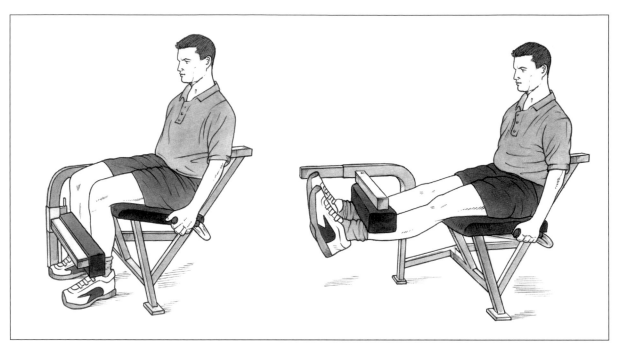

Above: To work your quadriceps, sit with your back straight and arms locked to your side. Raise the weight with your shins, until your legs are straight. Lower slowly and smoothly, and repeat.

If you are training for a particular sport, it is worth taking the time to identify which specific muscles you want to build in order to improve your performance. Swimmers, for example, will want to focus on shoulder and arm muscles, while runners may focus on legs. Do not forget, however, that you need a good foundation of overall strength on which to build, otherwise the body becomes unbalanced. We should also remember that those involved in military training programmes are open to a whole range of physical challenges, and it is difficult to train specifically for each one of them. In that case, a general weight training programme that builds overall strength will suffice.

Circuit Training

Circuit training is well suited to military training programmes as it improves strength while dovetailing well with other activities, such as running and swimming. The effect of circuit training is to strengthen your muscles and to increase the amount of muscle relative to fat in the body without an overall increase in body weight. Therefore, the weight you are carrying around is useful weight. The increase in muscle also means an increase in your body's metabolism, which means that fat is eaten up more quickly. Resistance training exercises, including circuit training, have the added benefit of reducing the risk of injury; they also help to improve body coordination and overall confidence. Most of all, of course, they build strength and stamina.

Circuit training is a mix of strength-building exercises that can be tailored to a specific sport or which provide an overall level of conditioning, the end result being that you will have more power to call on. As a general principle, you should have between six and 10 exercises in each circuit, and you should try to give a muscle group a rest after each exercise. In other words, after doing press-ups, for example, try an exercise that works out your legs. Make sure that you are fully warmed up before you attempt the exercises, and ensure that you warm down properly afterwards. You should repeat the circuit at least twice a week if you are working towards a military training programme or training for a high-impact event.

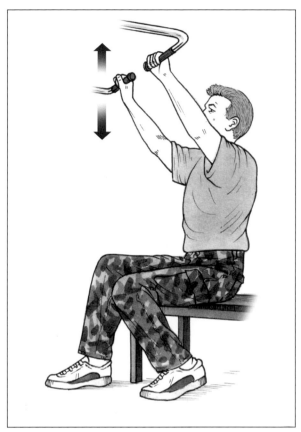

Above: For the shoulder press, hold the weight bar at shoulder level, then push it upwards. Lower it carefully and repeat. Perform three sets with rest periods of one minute between each set.

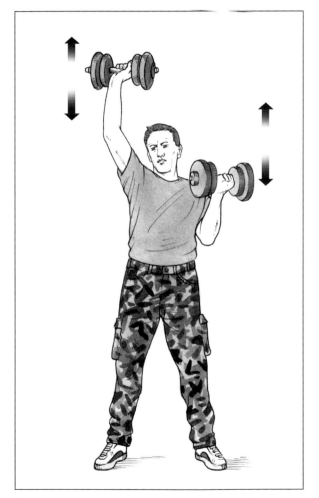

Above: For the barbell press, stand straight with your feet set slightly apart so that your weight is distributed evenly. Holding a barbell at the level of each shoulder, alternately raise them above your head.

The following are examples of typical military circuit training exercises, with advice as to their correct execution:

Press-ups: body forward over the shoulders, body weight supported on the hands; bend the arms at 90 degrees, then straighten them, keeping the body flat throughout; return to the first position.

Sit ups: lie flat on your back with knees bent and hands holding the back of your head; lift your torso at a 90-degree angle; lie back again until your shoulders touch the floor; your hands may be bent during the torso-raising process.

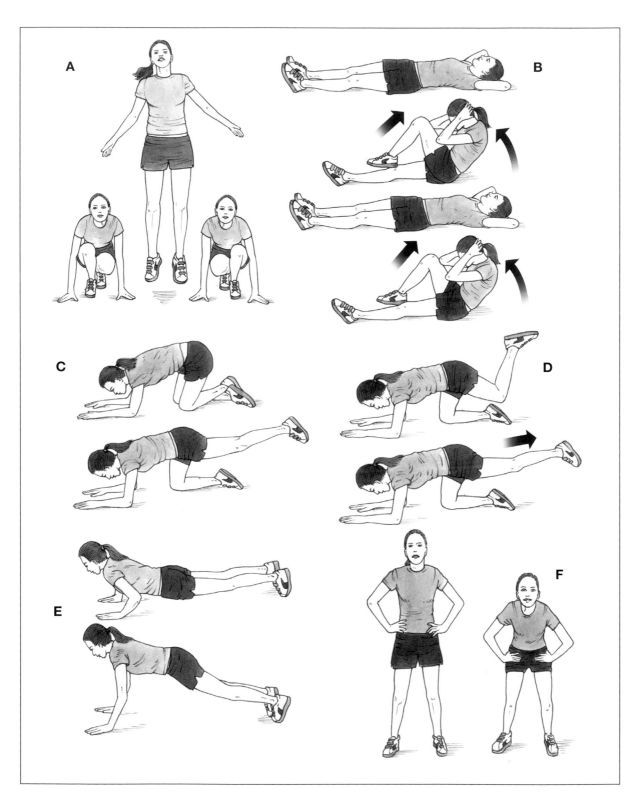

Burpees: stand upright, then bend your knees and descend into a squat position, with your hands on the ground; support your body weight on your hands, then push your legs back together, keeping your body straight, as if jumping into a press-up position; return your legs to the original position, with your knees under your chest; stand up and repeat.

Pull-ups: you need to hang from a bar with your feet clear of the ground; either jump up to the bar, to keep your feet clear, or bend your knees if the bar is lower so that your feet do not touch the ground; pull your body up with your arms until your chin is over the top of the bar; repeat.

Opposite: To perform this quick and easy circuit, repeat the following exercises:

A. Squat on the ground with right leg forward and left leg behind. Jump up and resume squatting position with left leg forward and right leg back. Repeat, then perform exercise with leg positions reversed.

B. Lie on the ground with your legs out straight and your hands clasped behind your head. Raise one leg and pull yourself up so that the opposite elbow touches the knee. Repeat on the other side.

C. Squat on the floor with your knees, elbows and forearms flat on the gound. Your left ankle should be wrapped over your resting right ankle. Keeping your back straight, slowly raise your left leg. Repeat with the other leg.

D. Squat on the floor with your knees, elbows and forearms flat on the gound. Keeping your back straight, kick out with your left leg and extend fully. Repeat with the other leg.

E. Press-ups: keep your back straight at all times and hands flat on the ground, shoulder-width apart. Bend your elbows until your chin touches the ground, then straighten them again – but do not lock elbows.

F. Place your hands on your hips and bend your knees to lower yourself before standing straight again. Keep your back straight throughout. Repeat 10 times.

Sprint: sprint to a point 60m (200ft) away, then jog back to the start; repeat.

Exercises should be alternated for best results: e.g. push-ups followed immediately by sit-ups, followed immediately by pull-ups – this way various muscles are tested. A variety of other exercises can be used in circuit training, according to the level of your fitness and physical development. The circuit might look something like this:

Suggested Circuit

WEEK	
1	• Press-ups x 7 • Sit-ups x 15 • Burpees x 10 (as fast as possible) • Pull-ups x 3 • You can do this circuit nonstop, then rest for a minute; perform the whole set three times over • At the end of the set, do 5 x 60m (200ft) sprints
2	• Press-ups x 10 • Sit-ups x 20 • Burpees x 12 (as fast as possible) • Pull-ups x 5 • Do full circuit three times, resting for a minute between each session; once you have completed all three circuits, do a 5 x 60m (200ft) sprint exercise once
3	• Press-ups x 12 • Sit-ups x 25 • Burpees x 15 (as fast as possible) • Pull-ups x 6 • Do full circuit three times, resting for a minute between each session; once you have completed all three circuits, do a 5 x 60m (200ft) sprint exercise once
4	• Press-ups x 15 • Sit-ups x 25 • Burpees x 18 (as fast as possible) • Pull-ups x 6 • Do full circuit three times, resting for a minute between each session; once you have completed all three circuits, do a 5 x 60m (200ft) sprint exercise once
5	• Press-ups x 20 • Sit-ups x 30 • Burpees x 21 (as fast as possible) • Pull-ups x 6 • Do full circuit three times, resting for a minute between each session; once you have completed all three circuits, do a 5 x 60m (200ft) sprint exercise once

United States Navy SEALs Suggested Physical Training Schedule I

WEEK	
1	• 4 x 15 push-ups • 4 x 20 sit-ups • 3 x 3 pull-ups
2	• 5 x 20 push-ups • 5 x 20 sit-ups • 3 x 3 pull-ups
3	• 5 x 25 push-ups • 5 x 25 sit-ups • 3 x 4 pull-ups
4	Ditto
5	• 6 x 25 push-ups • 6 x 25 sit-ups • 2 x 8 pull-ups
6	Ditto
7	• 6 x 30 push-ups • 6 x 30 sit-ups • 2 x 10 pull-ups
8	Ditto
9	• 6 x 30 push-ups • 6 x 30 sit-ups • 3 x 10 pull-ups

Opposite: Called an 'Oregon circuit', this circuit training programme originated in the United States, and is best performed outdoors:

A. Squat on the ground with right leg forward and knee tucked into the chest and left leg stretched behind. Jump up and resume squatting position with left leg forward and right leg back. Repeat, switching legs.

B. Lie on the ground with both knees bent and hands by your temples. Raise your back off the ground until your elbows touch your knees.

C. Lie on your back with both feet flat on the ground. Raise one leg and push it out straight. Repeat with the other leg.

D. To do press-ups, keep your back straight at all times and hands flat on the ground, shoulder-width apart. Lower your chest and chin towards the ground, bending from the elbows, then straighten them again – do not lock your elbows.

E. Stand with arms by your side. Jump up and simultaneously swing your arms up till your hands meet above your head. Repeat.

F. Lie on your back with hands behind your head. Raise one leg and pull yourself up, so that the opposite elbow touches the knee. Repeat on the other side.

G. Place your hands on your hips and bend your knees to lower yourself before standing straight again.

Treadmills

Place yourself in the press-up position, with both arms extended, then bring one leg up towards your chest, placing the ball of your foot on the ground. Do the same thing with the other leg, having returned the first leg to its original position. You should keep repeating the action rhythmically for a planned length of time.

Squat Thrusts

Stand with your arms at your sides, then squat down, placing both of your hands on the ground or floor. Shoot both legs backwards at the same time using a slight hop, until your legs are fully extended, then bring your knees immediately back up to your chest again. Continue repeating this exercise until a certain number of thrusts has been completed.

Crunches

Crunches can be a good way of strengthening the body for running, especially the ones that mimic the cross-over aspects of running motion, such as opposite arms and feet working together.

1. Basic crunch – Lie on your back with your knees bent, with both feet on the floor and hands behind your head. Using your stomach muscles, lift your shoulders slowly off the floor. Hold for about four seconds, then lower yourself back to the floor again.

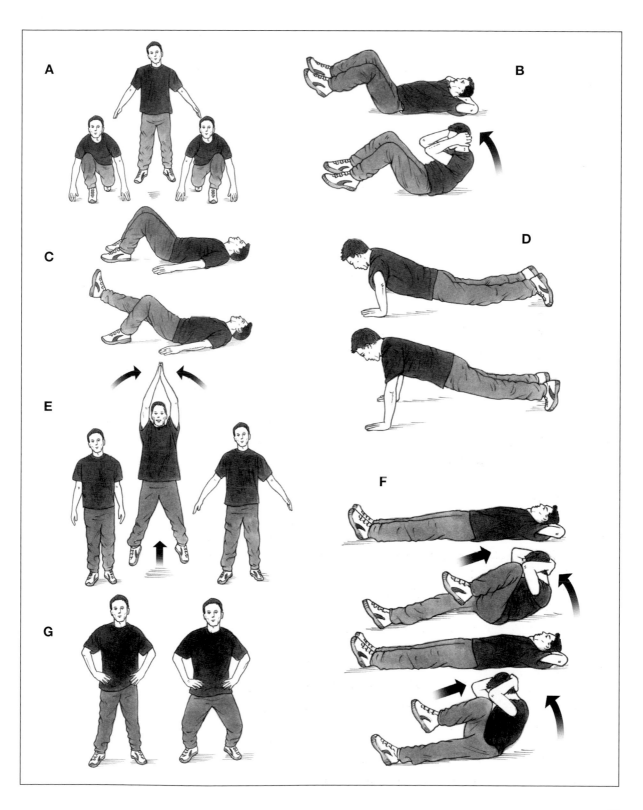

2. Side crunch – Lie on your back with your knees bent, both feet on the floor and hands behind your head. Now move one hand towards the foot on the same side, keeping the other hand behind your head. Repeat the exercise with the other hand.

3. The Bicycle – Lie on your back with your knees bent, with both feet on the floor and hands behind your head. Now bring each knee towards your chest and simultaneously twist the upper body and head round so that the elbow on the opposite side touches the knee. Repeat with the other knee and opposite elbow. Keep the straight leg in each case off the ground.

4. Reverse crunch – Lie on your back, then lift your legs until they are pointing straight up, at 90 degrees to the ground. Allow the small of your back to rest on the ground. Tighten and relax your stomach muscles.

Endurance Training

Many people will have experienced that humbling moment in a race, whether it is running, cycling, swimming or some other sport, when they know that they just do not have anything left. They can see the competitor in front of them, and they want to close the gap, or they can see the finish line and want to put in a final spurt before the opposition catches up with them, but they do not have the reserves of power. Such a moment is perhaps not the time to reflect on the differences between maximum strength, elastic strength and strength endurance, but these technicalities are central. Your maximum strength is the force that you are able to exert at any given moment on something like a heavy object, such as occurs during weightlifting. The maximum strength content of your performance tends to decrease as the longevity of the activity decreases.

The elastic strength of the muscles is shown in sports that require explosive energy, such as high jump or throwing a discus. Your endurance strength is defined by your ability to maintain a relatively high level of strength energy output over a period of time. This sort of strength is demonstrated in sprint rowing and some of the track events. It is well know that different sports train different muscles, and this knowledge can be used to develop a range of strength-training exercises that will make up for the limitations of a particular sport.

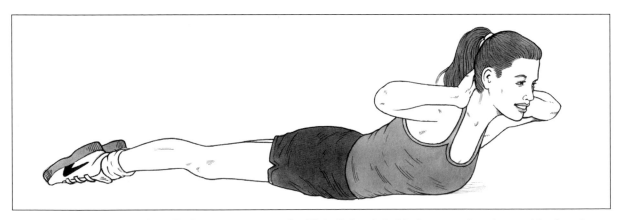

Above: To perform body raises, lie flat on your stomach with both hands behind your neck and your chin almost touching the ground. Slowly lift your chest off the ground and stretch backwards, before lowering yourself again to the almost-prone position. Repeat this exercise rhythmically for a set time or a set number of raises.

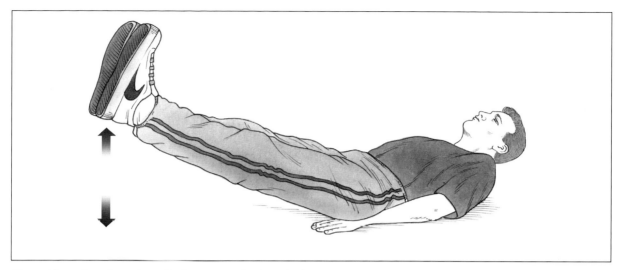

Above: To perform leg raises, lie flat on your back and raise your feet a few inches off the ground. Hold for a few moments, then lower. Repeat 10 times. You can also raise and spread your legs for variety.

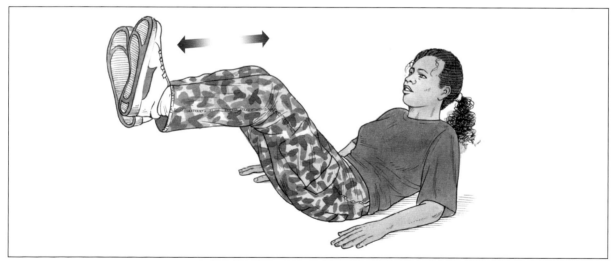

Above: To perform seated leg pushes, sit or lie on the ground with your forearms flat on the ground for support. Bring your knees up to your chest, then push your feet out above the ground until your legs are straight. Repeat.

Going back to the example of a runner, at the last stages of a race he or she would be delighted to find some extra power to put on a final spurt. A runner will not be able to find that power, however, if the muscles have not been developed through endurance training. Endurance strength can be built up by circuit training or hill running, for example. If you are destined for a military training course, you will greatly improve your chances of performing well by mixing in a wide variety of training exercises, each of which will condition different muscles in a different way, leaving you ready for anything, anytime, anywhere.

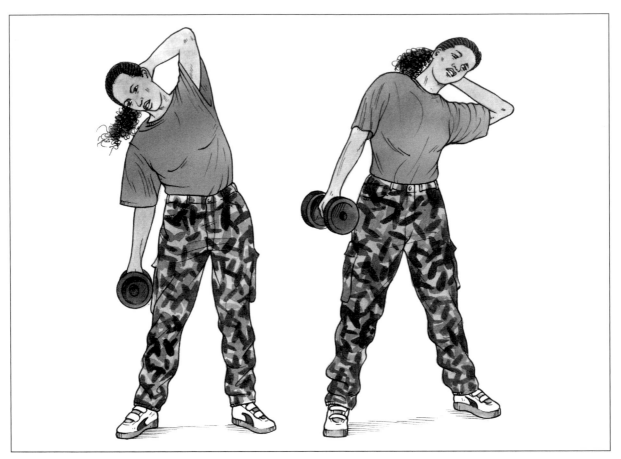

Above: Stand straight with one barbell by your side. Place one hand behind your head and lean over to the side of the barbell, then over to the other side. Repeat with the barbell in the other hand.

Endurance versus Strength Training

A widely accepted view has been that it is better to perform endurance training first, before working on strength training or speed work. The logic behind this is that you build a firm platform for more specific training. Widely accepted theories, however, eventually come under intense scrutiny and some research has been turning these ideas on their head, favouring explosive or strength training first, and moving on to endurance work. One issue raised is whether endurance and strength training are mutually compatible.

A study carried out in Canada in the 1980s, focusing on rowers, pitted two sets of athletes against each other. One group was tasked to perform five weeks of endurance work followed by five weeks of strength training, while the other group did the opposite. The results of the test, when measured in terms of lactate reduction and increased Vo2 max (the maximum rate of oxygen consumption), were surprisingly enough significantly in favour of the group which had done the strength, or circuit, training first.

The reasons for the advantage of strength training before endurance work is that stronger muscles have a greater resistance to fatigue than weaker muscles, and we should remember here that endurance training such as long runs do not necessarily make muscles bigger. A well-developed muscle does not have to work so hard, and therefore it tires less easily under strain. Athletes with strong muscles are more likely to have something left towards the end of their endurance phase, enabling them to keep going at a faster pace.

Another finding of the Canadian study was that those athletes who carried out the strength training before the endurance training did not tend to lose their strength during the endurance phase, even though they had stopped specific strength training.

Further studies have changed the mix of the training to make it less black and white: for example, they would mix running and strength training on the same day, with one coming before or after the other. When the training sessions were mixed together in this way, the results were less dramatic and tended to favour the traditional view that the endurance phase

should come first. One point that should be noted here is that a discipline such as running has the effect of warming up and conditioning the whole body, which puts it in the optimum state for the specific strength work. It is not such a good idea to go into a strength workout cold.

What conclusions can we draw from all this? First, the findings are not quite as revolutionary as they seem at first, and it all depends on how you mix your training regime. The research undertaken with groups doing entirely different exercise regimes for long periods showed that bigger and stronger athletes are better adapted to performing well in a long endurance session than their less-strong companions. The figures for Vo2 max will be higher simply because their muscles have greater capacity. On the other hand, endurance work does have an important part to play in warming up and conditioning the muscles, and an ideal exercise programme will combine both disciplines.

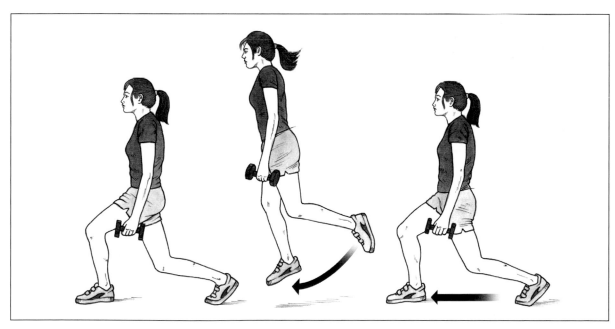

Above: With a barbell in each hand and your arms by your sides, place one leg forward and one leg back, bending at the knees. Jump up and cross your legs as you do so. Repeat 10 times.

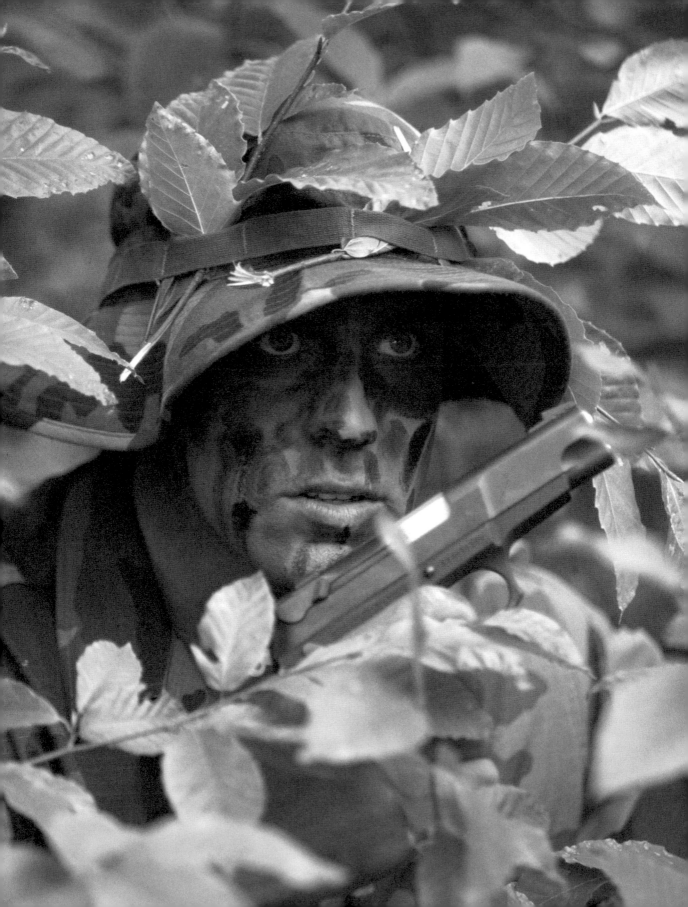

CHAPTER TWO

Mental Preparation

Once you have put together a consistent and varied physical training programme that you have resolved to follow faithfully, you are all set to go. You can feel yourself getting stronger; you are enjoying a sense of purpose.

Then fatigue kicks in, or you start to feel unwell. You have been overdoing it. That long run down the canal or through the park does not seem as inviting as it did three weeks ago. It is a chore to get down to the swimming pool when you are already pushed to fulfil all your other obligations and unexpected calls on your time. This was supposed to be fun; now it is a drag.

There is nothing so inviting and attractive as a gleaming well-defined goal. You can visualize it like the snow-capped Matterhorn on a sunny day and all the exhilaration you will feel when you conquer it. However, days, maybe weeks, later your enthusiasm begins to pall. The 'To Do' list seems to grow longer with each passing day. What had been fun and exciting has now turned into a slog. Time seems to be speeding away faster than you had allowed for.

Now is the time to revisit your goals. Despite the looming deadlines and the missed targets, you may have to stop, force yourself to take a rest, and review where you have got to. One of the simplest things that may need to be done is to review your milestones and targets, and make adjustments in order to make up for time lost due to unexpected commitments. Once you

Opposite: Keeping cool under pressure – mental training comes into its own when trying to evade an enemy force, whether on a training exercise or in a combat situation.

have taken it all apart and put it back together again in a manageable way you are likely to feel reinvigorated, even though there may now be more to achieve in a shorter space of time. You may also want to revisit your schedule. There are only so many hours in a day, but perhaps getting to bed a little earlier and getting into the habit of waking up earlier will help you to get more done. Maybe you should rearrange your plan of activities. Moving things around a bit will renew your sense of control and commitment. All this will help to stimulate a healthy attitude.

Ironing out the Flaws

On the face of it everything may seem OK. However, although there seems to be nothing

hindering your progress, and although you seem to be meeting your targets, there may come a point when you feel like a dog on a leash – suddenly pulled up. It can be the point where self-belief fails, where known experience runs out and the unknown begins, where self-doubt bites due to previous conditioning. Whatever the reason for reaching it, it is a point which has to be negotiated carefully or it may be a case of thus far and no further.

It may be just a small thing that is holding you back, but it can bring your dream crashing down if you do not deal with it. A bird may be held only by a thread, but it is enough to prevent it from flying. It may be pride that causes you to overlook some small detail. Military training

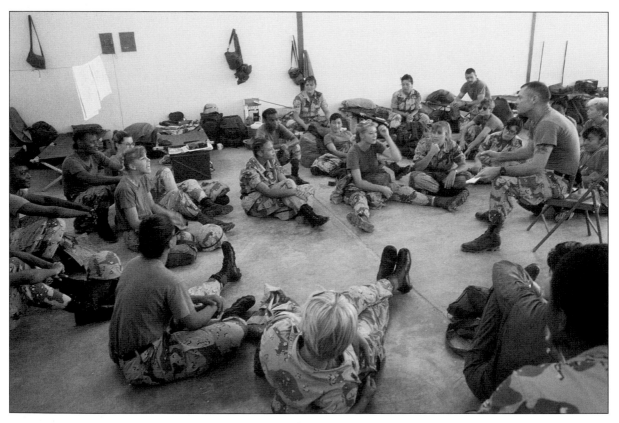

Above: Building teams involves an understanding of group psychology and how people relate to each other under stress. Here, a group of US soldiers discusses what went wrong in a recent training exercise.

programmes have a way of making sure that you remember that attention to detail is paramount. A piece of grit in your weapon could jam it when you and your buddies' lives depend on it. A pouch or button left undone could mean the loss of a vital piece of equipment.

Great men and great achievers often show both surprising humility and attention to detail, which probably partly explains how they became 'great' in the first place. Before the Battle of Fuentes de Onoro, May 1811, during the Peninsular War, the Duke of Wellington briefed his officers:

'It is to be hoped that the general and other officers of the army will at least acquire that experience which will teach them that success can be attained only by attention to the most minute details; and by tracing every part of every operation from its origin to its conclusion, point by point, and ascertaining that the whole is understood by those who are to execute it.'

This kind of approach resulted in the defeat of Napoleon Bonaparte, at that time the most powerful tyrant in Europe.

Part of a healthy mental attitude is to be confident that you have checked everything and that it is working, rather than leaving it to chance. This stimulates a healthy sense of self-reliance whereby you are less reactive, less a slave to rush and hurry, and less ready to rely on other people's opinions. Developing personal autonomy helps you to be more fully yourself, rather than playing a part. Sometimes people aspire to play a part for which they are not suited, which can be a sign either of pride or of a lack of confidence in their own abilities. Sometimes people act according to a script written by someone else, maybe a parent or significant other.

Understanding who you are, identifying your strengths and weaknesses (celebrating the first and coming to terms with the second), helps to make you a complete person and a stronger person because your energy is less likely to be dissipated chasing after unrealistic goals that are not suited to you.

A healthy self-knowledge also reduces the likelihood of another bad and damaging habit, namely the tendency to blame others when things go wrong. By knowing yourself and taking

GOALS

- Thoroughly review all the options; take advice where necessary before deciding on your goal.
- Check your goal is worthwhile.
- Plan out the short-term goals that will lead you to your ultimate goal.
- Visualize achieving the ultimate goal.
- Carefully focus on achieving each step on the way to the ultimate goal and make sure that you do everything well or to the best of your ability.
- Do not let worry about the size of the ultimate goal interfere with your attainment of shorter-term goals.
- Take time to plan realistic targets for achieving the shorter-term goals, being realistic about your time and any likely interruptions.
- Take time out from 'action' for 'visualization' of your goals.
- Tick off your achievements as you go, and learn from your mistakes.
- Resolve to pick yourself up and start afresh each new day. Persevere.

responsibility for your actions you possess your own life. Those who blame others are effectively placing their lives in other people's hands. You are responsible for what you think and feel, and the actions of others or the workings of chance should not change that.

Your life should be about action and not reaction. Some people are like balls in a pinball game, their destinies controlled by other people and events. A person who is self-controlled, aware of himself and conscious of his goals is better placed to deal calmly with the obstacles that life may throw at him. By taking care of the details and getting small things right you

gradually build up a foundation of confidence. Gradually your control over your environment will grow as you refuse to be distracted or rushed. You are no longer prey to chance circumstances or to the behaviour and attitudes of other people. By thinking for yourself, checking that what you say and think is really your opinion and not led by the desire to please or fit in, or that your thoughts were not put there by someone else, you foster a healthy self-reliant mental attitude.

Different people have different talents, and sometimes these talents are exceptional. However, even those with exceptional talents are

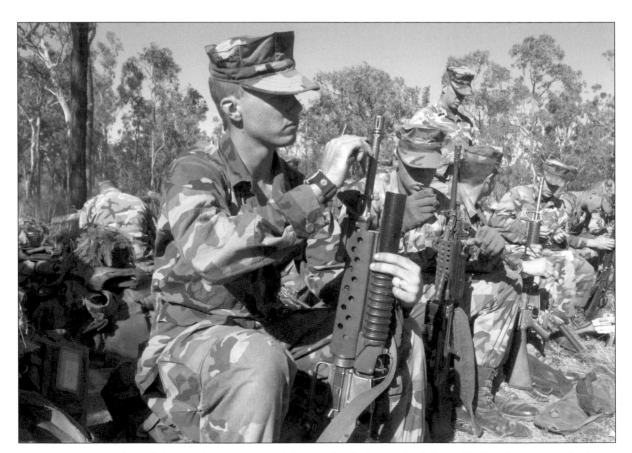

Above: US Marines clean their weapons before a training exerise in Queensland, Australia. Routine preparation is an essential part of teamwork which helps to build trust and confidence in a unit.

not immune from hard work. They do not spend their time purely in the glow of inspiration.

Wholeheartedness and Enthusiasm

Walter Chrysler, founder of Chrysler Motors, is recorded as saying that 'The real secret to success is enthusiasm.' Ralph Waldo Emerson said: 'Nothing great was ever achieved without enthusiasm.' So what is enthusiasm? The word actually means 'in God' or 'in a god' or 'to be inspired by a god'. The zeal of an enthusiastic person, therefore, is deemed to be otherworldly, even miraculous. This is because a truly enthusiastic person looks fired up, as if possessed, and seems to overcome obstacles in an almost supernatural way.

Enthusiasm can be personality related: gregarious extroverts probably make a better fist of outward enthusiasm than quiet introverts. You also have to watch out for hollow enthusiasm which seems incapable of analysing things in anything other than a positive light. If you have an extrovert boss and you happen to be an introvert, you will probably need to make extra effort to make your enthusiasm more visible. Extroverts are by definition people who have a strong filter against outside stimuli, so they need plenty of stimulus to make up for it. Introverts, on the other hand, have weak filters and take in plenty of stimuli, so they tend to want to quieten things down a bit.

Cheerfulness

Cheerfulness is similar to enthusiasm in that it requires effort and discipline to look on the good side of things. For the enthusiast and the cheerful person, the cup is definitely half full rather than half empty, and that is simply a result of changing their perspective. This positive outlook may take effort to begin with, but can soon become a habit.

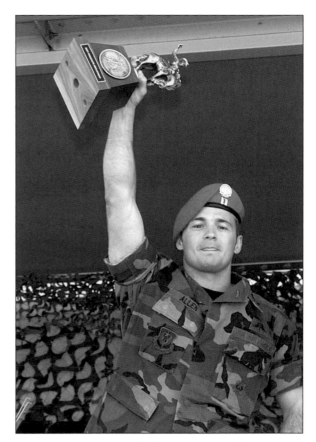

Above: Achieving goals is often the result of long-term planning, commitment and the ability to keep going, despite failures. Here, Captain Allen of the US Air Force's 320th Special Tactics Squadron hoists his first-place trophy for the Special Tactics Parachute Employment competition, 2000.

As with many qualities, cheerfulness is not necessarily felt so much as acted, at least at the outset. There may be many occasions when you feel genuinely cheerful, but a truly cheerful person remains so even when the going gets tough and there is no obvious light at the end of the tunnel.

Cheerfulness essentially involves looking at the good side of things and holding out the possibility of a positive outcome even when the going gets tough and the outlook looks

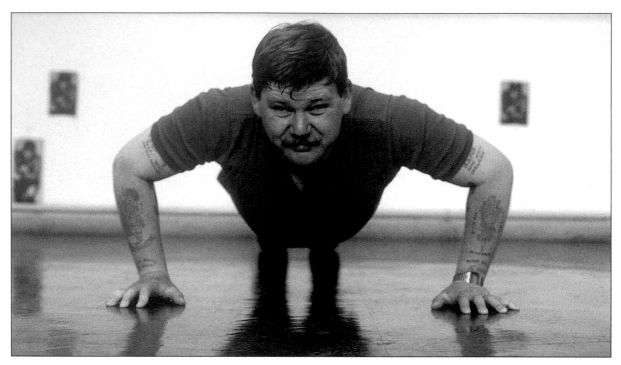

Above: Stress born of frustration can be expelled through vigorous physical exercise. Exercise produces endorphins, which create a natural sense of well-being.

bleak. It means providing a little sunshine even when there are grey clouds overhead.

A cheerful person is likely to have a few jokes to share even when it is pouring with rain and the trench you are standing in is half full of water. The cheerful person does not necessarily have to be the life and soul of the party, but his attitude should be informed by goodwill and patience. Depressing influences slide off the cheerful person like water off a duck's back. Cheerfulness is an outgoing attitude that helps others to cope, so a cheerful person is a real asset in any team. By being cheerful, you are more likely to forget your own problems and that stimulates creativity and helps you to cope.

Patience

Patience is the quality required to maintain internal stability in the face of obstacles, hard work and, more often than not, other people. The word is derived from the Latin word 'pati', to suffer, and whether you have to suffer cold, burdensome work or difficult people, by being patient you maintain your inner calm, self-control and judgment. By being patient you remain in control and do not become subject to other people's behaviour or the difficulties you may encounter.

Controlling Anger

There is only one thing to do with anger – get rid of it. You should treat anger as you would treat a loaded shotgun in a crowded place: pick it up carefully and unload it. The reason for this is that, although you may think that you use anger, in fact it uses you. Once the door is opened to anger, it just comes in and takes the place over. If anger takes you over, it is normally for the wrong reason: it may have something to do with fear, or panic or self-indulgence. This sort of anger can be readily distinguished from righteous anger, which is the positive reaction to some form of injustice, and which gives you the adrenalin and strength to defend yourself or others. When anger is allowed in, it tends to bring with it its own system of logic to replace the normal reasoning system you use when you are calm. In this way it is rather like a computer virus: it comes in, takes over and sends out abusive e-mails to all of your contacts. Anyone who is angry has an inflated and inflamed sense of their own point of view, and reason goes right out of the window.

Once you decide to do without anger, a whole new set of options present themselves for dealing with difficult people and difficult circumstances. The difference is, this time you will be in control through the exercise of proper reason. You will have more time to consider things and to judge your responses, rather than shooting from the hip and getting yourself embroiled in all sorts of difficulties. Not getting angry about some injustice does not mean being passive or a doormat. The difference is that anger is a reaction, whereas a calm and reasonable response is action.

When you hold on to resentment or anger, you may think you are doing something about an annoying circumstance and that your anger shows you are rejecting the thing or person who has annoyed you. In fact, the opposite is the case. Being angry with someone has been compared to putting your hands round his throat – his face is always before you. By constantly turning over an annoying comment in your mind or thinking about other people's annoying attitudes, you are in fact allowing these things to affect your thinking. Also, despite the complexity of the human mind, it is not good at

EMOTIONS AND MOODS

- Do not allow your plans to be altered by what you 'feel' or by chance events.
- Successful people remain consistent, despite difficulties.
- Place a positive perspective on everything that happens.
- Control any negative moods before they escalate and control you.
- Give yourself time for rest and recreation so that you return both refreshed and strengthened to the task in hand.
- Remember your achievements and celebrate them.
- Put the past behind you.
- Learn to remain calm and in control.

thinking of more than one thing at any one time: if you are thinking about a negative event, you do not have any space to think of something positive. Annoyances are like mosquito bites – the more you scratch them, the more inflamed they get. The best thing to do is just leave them alone. Annoying thoughts, however, also need to be replaced by something more positive; in other words, if there is any empty space, something has got to fill it. If you fill the space with positive, calm, reasonable thoughts, there will be no room for negative ones.

Anger has physical effects due to the in-built fight or flight response. When you hold on to anger, your adrenalin is released and your muscles are powered ready for action. If there is no release of this energy, it just puts a strain on your system and becomes stress. Constant stress is bad for the body and you may also end up with stomach problems, as anger tends to create inflammation of the stomach lining that can lead to ulcers.

MEDITATION

Meditation is an art that can help you to focus more clearly on your goals and to discard distractions.

As your mind is often filled with plans and mental activity, it will come as a shock if you try to stop it and focus on one thing or try to achieve total internal silence. This will take practice and patience.

- Find a quiet place where you can be alone.
- Sit comfortably with your back straight, and make sure you will not be distracted.
- Breathe regularly and deeply, and slow down your physical and mental tempo.
- Stop your mind planning or worrying about past or future events, and focus on a particular word or phrase. Alternatively, you could focus on a picture.
- Try to still your mind and keep focusing on the word or image for about 10 minutes. As distracting, busy thoughts come into your mind, let them go.

Over the next days and weeks, gradually lengthen the time of your meditation session, up to 30 or 45 minutes.

With practice, you should find that your ability to focus improves and that you develop greater control over your mental activity. This helps to give more force to your decisions and actions.

Meditation and Calm

Calmness has been identified as a recurrent characteristic of natural leaders. If there is a crisis, people naturally turn to a calm person who is able to maintain his reason and judgment, size up what needs to be done and give instructions. Calmness can be cultivated; one of the ways to do this is through meditation.

To refocus and re-anchor yourself through meditation, you need to take time away from plans and activities, and as far as possible step outside the normal run-of-the-mill pattern of life. For example, there is the story of the bearers in a jungle who were sitting down on a march replied when challenged that they were waiting for their souls to catch up. Forward momentum and activity can become a drug, and can result in a loss of direction and motivation.

The other advantage of meditation is that it tends to put an end to some of the negative self-talk that can drag us down. We tend in meditation to, like the bearers in the jungle, unhitch the baggage we often carry around with us and take a rest. Somehow we feel liberated, even if only for a while, and discover something of our essential being. The more practise we get at this, the more free we are likely to be, although it would be naive to think we can just walk off for the rest of the journey and leave all the luggage behind.

However, on some expeditions, a decision sometimes need to be made about thinning down the load, otherwise you might never reach the final destination. This is a good opportunity to get rid of that baggage which includes the negative influences you have picked up in life, due to other people's problems, limitations and weaknesses. The luggage you still have to take represents all the difficulties and challenges that we invariably encounter in life, but the burden is less now, partly because your attitude is now

Right: The benefits of meditation have been appreciated for centuries. Meditation can help to improve your focus and your self-control.

changed and you are not weighed down by the excess baggage.

The essence of meditation is to calm the mind and concentrate on one word or phrase, or even an image. The point is to cut out the normal chatter that fills our minds and let the image, word or image gradually become the focus. Meditation can be practised in short periods throughout the day or in single longer sessions, such as half an hour to an hour. It will probably take practise to build up to longer periods of meditation, and it is important to persist.

The effect of meditation, apart from burning away some of the negative dross that may be burdening your subconscious, is to make your day calmer and better ordered. By stopping the flow of action you effectively stop the clock for a while and bring time under control. Once you have done this it will seem less as if time is running through your fingers. It may be that when you are out on a trail run or on a bike you dash past some beautiful view out over the landscape. Why not walk out to that spot and take in the view, focusing on it for its own sake. As we are essentially part of nature, getting into nature is a good way of meditating, calming things down and putting things in perspective.

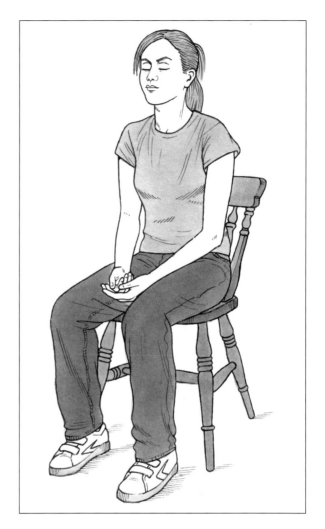

Self-Esteem

Much has been written on the subject of self-esteem, and it has become something of a buzz phrase. As with many buzz phrases, however, people tend to turn their thought processes off and not ask what it actually means. Low self-esteem is usually taken to mean that you feel bad about yourself or your achievements. In order to raise your self-esteem, some experts

seem to say, you have to tell yourself that you are a good person and reverse the negative process. The problem with this is that, if you have a low opinion of yourself, what difference will it make if you yourself start telling yourself that you are all right.

Religious people solve this problem by looking outside themselves and thanking God for the wonder of their being. So the religious perspective is not about self-esteem at all: it is about God's esteem for you as part of His creation. The advantage of this is that it places you outside the sphere of the negative people around you who may have affected your self-esteem and sense of self-worth.

Gaining your own approval or other people's approval as a means of raising your self-esteem can produce problems because you may find yourself reacting to their limited viewpoint and wasting your time and your talents. If someone decides to annoy you by suggesting you are no good in some way, you may set out to prove them wrong in order to raise your self-esteem. In fact, what they are referring to may not be where your talents lie, so if you react to their comments you could engage in a great deal of effort with limited results. Once you have reached the point where you can 'prove' them wrong, they will probably just ignore you because their initial criticism was based on some kind of jealousy or insecurity of their own. It is better to just walk away from negative comments and negative people and try to think clearly about what you are good at, not allowing yourself to be controlled by the expectations of others.

Another notion that is often peddled by the self-esteem lobby is that you cannot love others unless you love yourself. This again needs to be subjected to scrutiny. We should accept that we are all a mixture of good and bad and that we need to try to focus on the good in ourselves, as well as the good in others. We do not need to wait for eternity until we have discovered that we

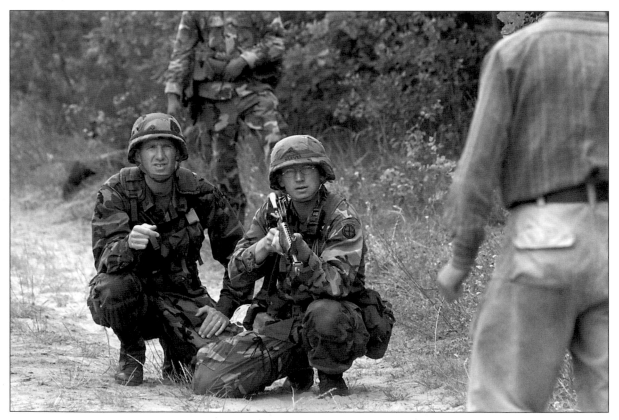

Above: Here, in a role-play scenario, a US soldier negotiates with a potential civilian assailant. Body language can be altered according to the level of threat. These soldiers are ready to act, but their stance is essentially interrogative and open. By crouching down, they have made themselves both a smaller target and less threatening.

are all good before appreciating others. In fact, the opposite is the case. By accepting our own faults, we are in a far better position to accept the faults of others.

Service

Anyone who signs up for a military training programme is entering a service. He is not there for himself, but there to perform a service for others, and in the military that can mean putting your life on the line. Although there may be a great deal of individual competitiveness in military training programmes, there is always a team element. Even gold medallists at the Olympics, although they have achieved something as individuals, are also representatives of a team and a country.

If you feel you have to win all the time, if beating people is a preoccupation, you may need to change your attitude. On a military training course you may be the first back – you have beaten the opposition and by the time the rest come in you may have already showered and changed, and be into your second helping of dessert. Then you notice something. The person you considered to be your chief competitor for first place is coming in with the also-rans, but he seems strangely cheerful and popular. Then the CO walks in and goes over to his table. He seems to be congratulating him. You were the one who came first. Why is he not congratulating you?

It turns out that your competitor came upon someone who had hurt his leg during the run. He stayed with this person, encouraging and supporting him until the next checkpoint, when the wounded man could be put on a vehicle. He did a good job of making up some of the lost time, but he was well behind his expected performance. To add insult to injury, the CO had been watching the whole thing from the top of a nearby hill.

So there are different types of winning. One is the worldly feeling you get when you beat others and confirm how good you are, and the other is about living up to your principles and thinking of others. Military training programmes are about

KEEP CALM UNDER STRESS

One of the most decisive factors for passing or failing an elite forces soldier is his ability to cope with pressure and stress. You may have the ability, the physical strength and the intelligence to deal with physical and mental challenges, but if you lose your cool under pressure you will go no further.

Shouting and anger are signs that you are losing control. You may be able to force others to do what you want, but in the process you will lose their respect and they will no longer regard you as a natural leader.

Practise remaining calm in stressful situations, particularly when you are tired, and try to think clearly. Keep your options down to a minimum, especially when you are tired and find it difficult to concentrate.

Once you have made a decision, follow it through in a calm and determined way, blocking out negative thoughts or criticism from others with positive affirmations.

Even if your decision may not have been the best one, your determination can turn it into the right one in the end.

individual achievement and endurance, but they are also about teamwork, about people who are not only good, but who can also help their buddies. A military unit can move only as fast as its slowest member, and to function properly everyone needs to be looking out for his comrade. This principle does not mean, of course, that you have to treat others as if they cannot manage themselves, it just means providing the right level of encouragement and support when necessary.

Confidence

Confidence is rooted in two Latin words meaning 'with' and 'trust'. Doing things with confidence means doing them with the trust that they will work out. It means performing tasks in a wholehearted, committed way unencumbered by self-doubt or wavering. It is a quality that is expected of servicemen and women.

The benefits of confidence are manifold, for confident action almost invariably elicits a positive response from others. The other benefit is that confidence places us positively in new realms of experience, allowing us to gain more confidence to handle new environments, which in turn empowers us to move forward again.

Unfortunately, confidence is not easy to acquire, unless you already have it. However, although you may not feel confident about something, if you act confidently you may find your way into reaping all the benefits enjoyed by confident people. Acting confidently means going through all the motions that a confident person would use, acting with self-belief, behaving in an open, determined way, thinking about your achievements, looking at the constructive aspects of any feedback, positive or negative, and acting with courage and determination. If you make this act a habit, you may find that the role you are playing becomes an intrinsic part of your personality and that you have left behind self-doubt, wavering and timidity for ever.

Just as you cannot expect to take part in a play without first learning your lines, you cannot expect to act confidently or, even less, be confident without some preparation. You have to set yourself up for success by doing adequate preparation, rather than setting yourself up for failure by skating over essentials. Part of this process is to learn from your mistakes. Some

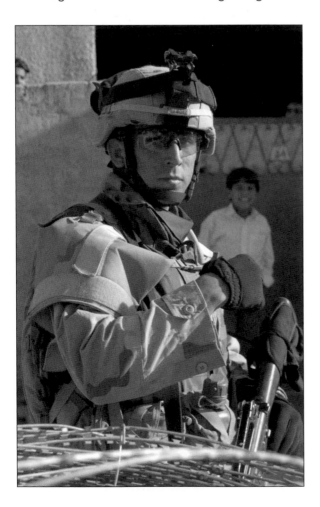

Left: The military life presents men and women with constant challenges. In meeting and overcoming them, confidence is born. Here, a US soldier carries out a routine patrol in Baghdad, March 2005.

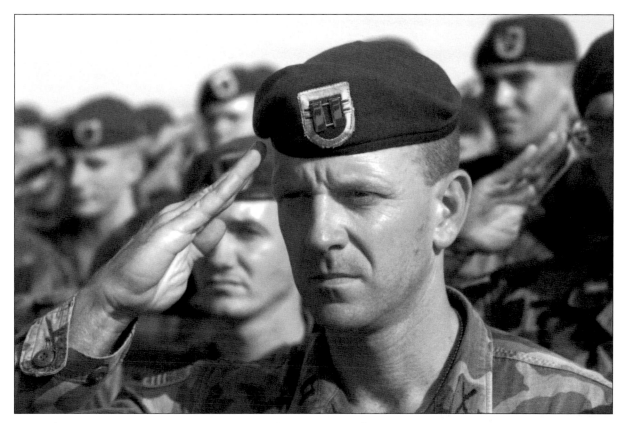

Above: Soldiers are not machines; they are human beings. They do, however, have to be able to accept duty and discipline without question, even to the point of laying down their lives.

people grind along in the slow lane because they have not learned from and adapted to past experiences. The more time you take to identify negative experiences and learn to avoid them, the less likely they are to crop up on you when you are least expecting it or to influence your behaviour in ways you cannot pin down.

You may need to note down previous incidents in which you exhibited behaviours you want to change. They may have something to do with the timing of a comment in a meeting, or your decision to move up a gear in a race. If you experience a negative feeling about your ability to perform, you may want to consider why that is. Either keep moving forward to prove yourself wrong, or rationalize how a similar circumstance

may have met with negative result in the past. Then either go forward or take further time to train and prepare.

Gaining confidence may be compared to going through a series of watersheds. We are pushing back the boundaries of our experience, and this involves a certain amount of walking into the unknown. We need to steel ourselves before each advance, drawing as much as possible on our previous experience and using the information in a constructive way.

Each person is unique and therefore there are situations that affect your confidence which do not trouble the next person. If there is a particular group dynamic that invariably leaves you worse off, where your ideas are not

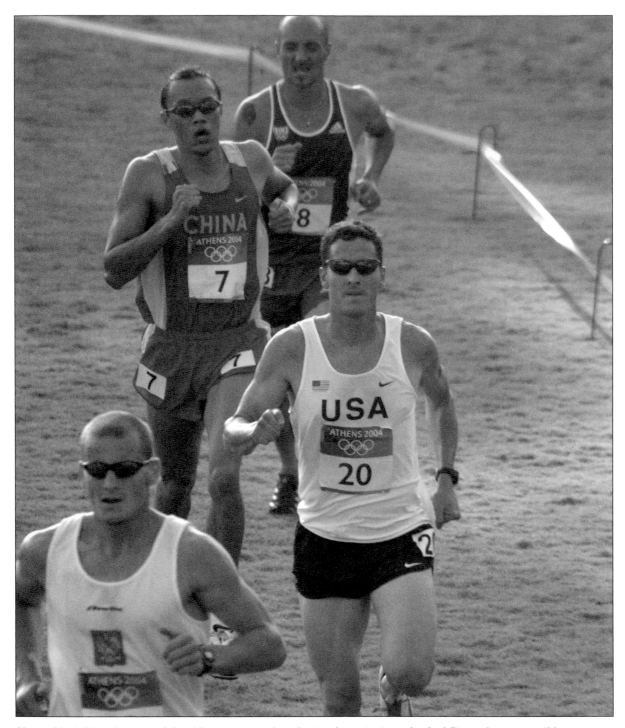

Above: Mental toughness and the drive to succeed are just as important as physical fitness in a competitive environment. Here, US 1st Lieutenant Chad Senior (number 20) pulls for the finishing line in the Men's Pentathlon at the 2004 Olympics in Athens, Greece.

acknowledged, for example, this is a scenario that will damage your confidence. Either you have to protest about it or you need to untangle yourself from it because other people will be benefitting at your expense. It may be, however, that if you were to put forward the same ideas to a different group in different circumstances you and your ideas will be greatly appreciated. There is a whole host of incidents and attitudes that can put you off your stride and diminish your performance, including other people, the weather, work schedules and so on. The difference between high-level performers and also-rans is that the latter allow themselves to be put off by all these factors, while the former focus on their inner strength and go on regardless. To gain confidence we need to approach things with a can-do attitude, and this is much more likely to produce results than if we were to take a hesitant or negative attitude.

Another trick is to be more relaxed with yourself and with others. Do not to burden yourself with expectations that you will find difficult to meet. Although you need to prepare yourself well in order to be and appear competent, and to enable a positive outcome, you have to make allowances for the occasional glitches. If you are going to make a presentation and the slide projector does not work, you cannot allow this to throw you off balance. You need to approach the problem in a relaxed way. The more anxious you get, the more restricted your blood flow, which literally means less oxygen getting through to the brain. A confident person does not act as if there is someone holding a stopwatch. Confident people always seem to have plenty of time in hand. They can pause to think carefully about something, and their delivery is not hurried. Confident people do not keep glancing nervously at the audience to see if there is any positive feedback on the faces of the audience, only to discover that there is not and thereby become even more nervous. A confident person imposes his sense of well-being on others; he does not depend on their feedback to make him feel good.

Projecting Confidence

If you are in a meeting or giving a presentation and you feel tense, this tension is communicated in your voice. A feeling of constriction and over-breathing can make your voice sound more highly pitched than usual. One way to counteract this is to control your breathing. If you breathe deeply and slowly, taking each breath into the bottom of your stomach, you should feel calmer and maintain the normal timbre of your voice.

Public speakers are invariably tempted to talk too fast and, once they are up on the podium, the slightest pause can seem like an age. It is, however, important to learn to dwell on significant words and to use pauses for effect in order to maintain the audience's attention. If you become more involved with what you are saying and think about the meaning of the words, any worries you may have about your audience should dissipate.

Words are associated with meaning. The more we can imaginatively connect ourselves with the meaning of words, the better we will project what we are trying to say and the less worried we will be about the reaction. We can often see ourselves negatively by projecting our negative thoughts about ourselves on to others. If we get it into our heads that certain people have negative impressions of us, then we can tend to look for evidence to back it up. If someone makes a chance remark that happens to fit our negative self-perspective, we might easily take that as 'proof' and even give them a hard time, when they actually meant nothing of the sort. If you have secure, confident thoughts about yourself, then you are more likely to project those thoughts on to others and gain positive feedback.

In military training, a soldier is required to both take and give criticism. There will be plenty of taking in such training, not all of which is

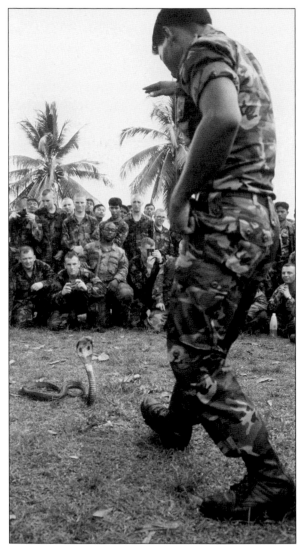

Above: Elite forces acquire exceptional skills in handling the rigours and dangers of the natural world. Here, a Thai special forces soldier demonstrates how to cope with a cobra.

designed to be reasonable or balanced! However, as the soldier moves on in his career he will become aware of certain basic principles: an officer should never criticize another officer in front of the men, and non-commissioned officers should observe the same rules. As far as possible, criticism should be mixed with encouragement – in other words, it should be constructive, and also to the point. In your own sphere of activity, remember to criticize other people's behaviour and not their personalities or anything else they cannot change. Try to end on a positive note, with positive suggestions for improvement. Do not become emotionally involved: if you are angry or if you dislike the person concerned, it will be difficult to offer impartial criticism.

Self-Knowledge

Self-knowledge is about knowing who you are and what you are good at and this plays an important role in building confidence. You need to sit down and check what you are good at and the sort of roles to which you are suited. Then you need to analyse the roles you are currently playing and see if they match with your talents. If they do not match it may be because you are playing roles devised by others and conforming too much to others' expectations.

This process can, of course, be taken too far. It may be that you have a job that is not intrinsically interesting, but which fulfils the requirement of providing you and your family with a reasonable income. Such a situation may in turn empower you to engage in leisure pursuits which you find rewarding. If your job, however, is inherently unsuitable, you may not be performing as well as you might elsewhere, and it could be time to revisit your goals.

Having a better knowledge of yourself, of your individual tastes and skills, can help to boost confidence because you come to appreciate your individuality and the particular gifts you have to offer. This realization goes hand in hand with cultivating the habit of thinking carefully about what other people say and judging your individual reaction and opinion, rather than just jumping on to the bandwagon. Very often we say things because we are eager to please someone else or because we are afraid of disagreeing with them. Thinking carefully about your own views can help you to break free from these constraints. Strangely enough, the negative reaction we sometimes get from people when we express our own opinions can be very liberating, as it is a sign that we have broken out of the circle of their expectations and have become more fully ourselves.

The path to self-knowledge involves identifying whether you are an extrovert or an introvert, and what sort of skills you apply to problems. These aspects of your personality can best be identified by taking personality tests, such as the Myers Briggs test.

Body Language

Your body language will often say more about you than what you say. An estimated 65 per cent of messages are sent non-verbally, and so physical traits have a huge influence on how we are assessed and judged. Although body language is frequently spoken of in reference to interview skills and office presentations, it also has a major impact in the military field, as a soldier is more often than not seen, rather than heard. A Guardsman with inadequate body language would stick out a mile on Horse Guards Parade, as would a marine with a similar attitude on duty outside the White House. Confidence and self-respect expressed in body language matter a great deal. Soldiers are also expected to be open and assertive in their gaze.

A soldier's body language is not rigid, unless on parade, and the movements are fluid, expressive of a fit and well-conditioned body. The head position is level, and the hands are kept away from the face.

Physical exercise improves your posture, and it can be a good idea to exercise before making a presentation. First, it tends to smooth out any

POSITIVE THINKING

● Get into the habit of thinking that the glass is half-full, not half-empty.

● Look for the good side of everything – even when it is raining.

● Listen carefully for and challenge negative or anxious thoughts.

● Do not personalize failure, but take an objective view of the circumstances.

● If things do not work out as you would have wanted, take an objective inventory of what you might do differently and better next time.

● Do not use failure to 'prove' you are unworthy; remain cheerful in difficult circumstances.

● Become comfortable with the idea of success.

● Do not expect approval from others and have the courage to continue regardless.

● Recognize you cannot control or change other people's attitudes and reactions.

● Remember that you control your own thoughts and emotions, and do not give that power to anyone else.

● Take time to reaffirm positive thoughts until they become habitual and ingrained.

● Keep things in proportion.

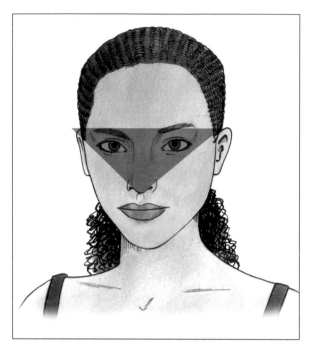

Above: The 'eye-nose triangle' is the area of the face you should focus on for 65–70 per cent of the time. Looking either above or below this area can have negative connotations.

potential muscle twitches; secondly, it helps your breathing, making it deeper and your voice more resonant; and, thirdly, it clears your throat, sinuses and other passageways. You can also go through a routine of face massage, by making exaggerated smiles, raising your eyebrows and moving your mouth from side to side. This activity tones the many facial muscles, making it easier to smile when necessary.

Eye Contact

If you were a soldier, standing to attention on parade, and a colour sergeant was politely advising you that you need to stand closer to your razor during your morning shave, there is one thing you must not do if you plan to complete your training course – look him in the eye. Army recruits learn very quickly about eye contact: when speaking to an NCO or officer they will normally look straight at the cap badge, if they want to be spared 50 press-ups or a 'beasting' round the parade ground.

In more normal circumstances, eye contact can be developed so as to make the best impression and to facilitate conversation. There are optimum target areas in the face that you should look at, as well as areas you should try to avoid. The way we look at someone tells them a great deal about our attitude and tends to elicit a proportionate reaction. The recruit may have no choice other than to stare at the cap badge, the NCO is likely to be staring unblinkingly at the eyes and face of the recruit. This demonstrates that the NCO is in a dominant position. If the recruit were to stare back, it would be taken as a sign of insolence, or daring to suggest that he is on equal terms with the NCO. Such an affront would invariably result in a lot more physical exercise for the recruit than he had anticipated.

Where two people are exchanging conversation on equal terms, the eye contact will tend to be moderate and equal. Too much staring would suggest either an argument or aggression, and too little eye contact or looking down would suggest that one person in the conversation is submissive to the other. If you tend to look away from someone who is talking to you, it probably indicates that you are not interested in them or in what they are saying. A measured, direct and open gaze is likely to give the other person the impression that you are receptive to what they are saying, and the same rule works the other way round. If, on the other hand, you look at people warily and try to avoid eye contact, or maintain a frown, you will quickly give them the impression that you do not like them and they are likely to respond in kind.

In general, your body language will betray what you are thinking and what your attitudes are. It is easy to tell the difference, for example, between a false smile and a genuine one. So if you want to have positive body language, try to think in a positive, fearless way. It can also work the other way round: if you make an effort to smile, uncross your arms and your legs, and act in a more open and relaxed way, your mind can often take its cue from the physical behaviour and you will therefore feel more relaxed and confident. Physical exercise and strength will have an influence on this, as will the self-respect

that comes from self-discipline, achievement and teamwork.

If you are in front of a group of people, you may be inclined to restrict your eye contact to the person who is talking with you, but try to take in as many others of the group as possible. When speaking either to an individual or a group, maintain as much eye contact as you would when listening. By looking at them, you back up what you are saying. If you do not look at them, they are likely to value your comments less.

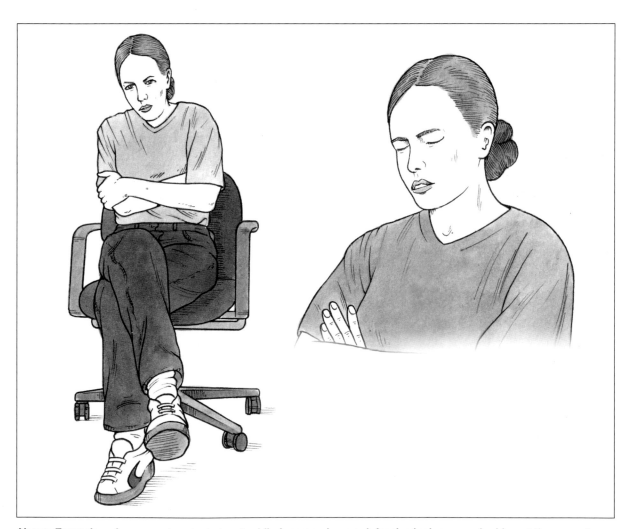

Above: Examples of poor posture include a huddled, crossed-arms defensive look or eyes looking at the ground. This almost always gives a negative impression.

It is quite difficult to focus on both eyes at once, where this is appropriate. If you get into the habit of moving between the eyes of the other person, it reduces the effect of staring, makes you seem more interested and intelligent, and gives the person the positive feedback that you are listening very carefully to whatever it is that they are saying.

Courage

Courage is related to confidence, and it involves facing our fears and overcoming them. Courage and fear are intimately related – two sides of the same coin. A person who is not afraid is not a courageous person. Courage is always to do with overcoming the instinct to turn back or not go forward through fear of the consequences, which may involve physical or mental hardship.

Some people are more predisposed to anticipate potential outcomes than others, and what it may require courage for one person to do may be something that another would have no trouble with. Some people are so thick-skinned that they do not even notice the things that cause fear to others. Courage is exercised by the will and enables us to overcome fear and to

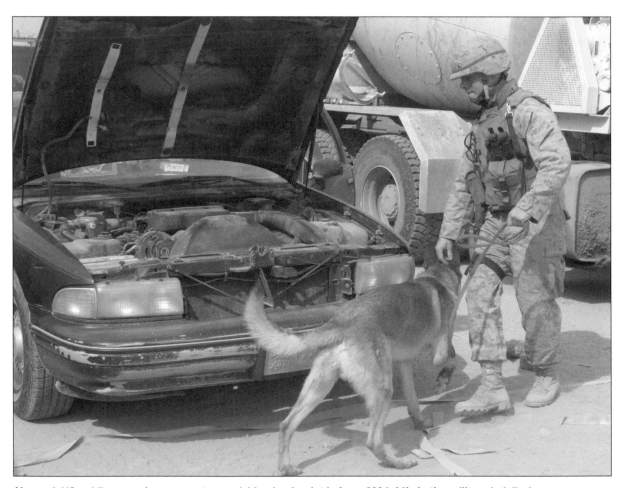

Above: A US soldier searches a car at a roadside checkpoint in Iraq, 2004. Life in the military is full of unseen dangers. You are an ideal target for those who want to make a political point.

COMMITMENT

In his novel *David Copperfield*, considered to be the most autobiographical of his works, Charles Dickens put the notion of commitment this way:

'I will only add, to what I have already written of my perseverance at this time of my life, and of a patient and continuous energy which then began to be matured within me, and which I know to be the strong part of my character, if it have any strength at all, that there, on looking back, I find the source of my success. I have been very fortunate in worldly matters; many men have worked much harder, and not succeeded half so well; but I never could have done what I have done, without the habits of punctuality, order, and diligence, without the determination to concentrate myself on one object at a time, no matter how quickly its successor should come upon its heels, which I then formed. [...] My meaning simply is, that whatever I have tried to do in life, I have tried with all my heart to do well; that whatever I have devoted myself to, I have devoted myself to completely; that in great aims and in small, I have always been thoroughly in earnest. I have never believed it possible that any natural or improved ability can claim immunity from the companionship of the steady, plain, hard-working qualities, and hope to gain its end. [...] there is no substitute for thorough-going, ardent, and sincere earnestness. Never to put one hand to anything, on which I could throw my whole self; and never to affect depreciation of my work, whatever it was; I find, now, to have been my golden rules?'

move forward to accomplish a difficult task. Once exercised, courage helps to increase confidence, so that if you face your fear in one area you may then move on to dominate your fear in other areas.

One way of overcoming fear with courage is to act energetically, though not rashly, and not to argue with fear. The more we consider the fearful consequences of some action, the more likely we are to be paralysed by it. Courage involves to some extent ignoring the voice of fear so that the will to act and to move forward predominates.

Fear is a safety mechanism and should be listened to when judging an action. It is not courageous but foolish to put your life at risk unnecessarily. There may be perfectly rational reasons why you think you cannot do something, as it may be something of which you have little or no experience. The root of some fear can be the unknown and we have to steel ourselves to have faith that we can overcome despite our lack of experience.

As with many other virtues, courage rarely means feeling brave; it is more to do with acting bravely: hence the title of the bestselling book: *Feel the Fear and Do it Anyway* by Susan Jeffers. To demonstrate courage, you have to act as if you were not afraid at all. The courage usually has to come from within ourselves, although others may encourage us. If we do not exercise courage to overcome our fear in one direction, it may well influence our decision in another direction, so that gradually we become hemmed in by our fears and unable to function. If that happens, we need to break out of the ring of fears so that we can realize our potential.

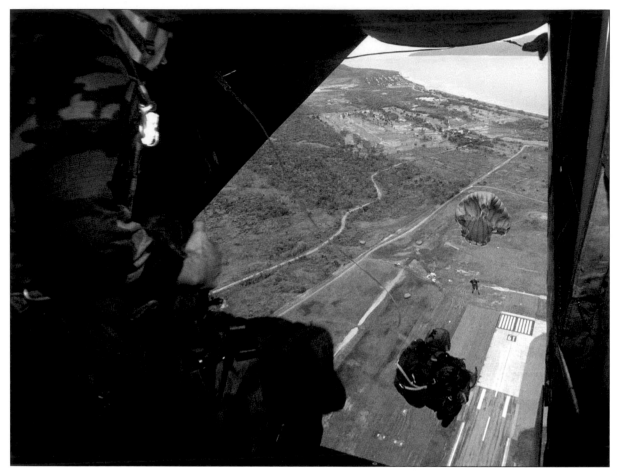

Above: Jumping out of an aeroplane involves a large measure of trust in your training and in your equipment. It also requires courage in the face of fear.

Real courage is often associated with duty – in other words, things that we know we are supposed to do, but are disinclined to. Courageous people are not necessarily fired up or inflamed with passion. In fact, people who are angry and noisy, or who bully, are often people who are disguising fear, confusion or inadequacy. Carrying out a difficult duty is often associated with calm and serenity because courage involves centring the forces required for forward movement into danger and the unknown. Courageous action may sometimes involve going 'over the top' into a hail of machine-gun fire, but often the best way to demonstrate courage is through assured and deliberate action. A frenzy of energy may seem like courage at the time, but it is also more likely to dissipate, like a balloon that blasts crazily around a room until all the air runs out and it falls limply to the ground.

Discouragement is the greatest enemy of courage. One of the effects of discouragement is to make you think that you are too late, or that you have messed something up, or perhaps that someone else is doing it better. You may also have someone telling you that you cannot do it and blocking your way. Again, by putting together a plan of action and calmly beginning to carry it out, you disprove the internal or external voices of discouragement and gradually begin to move forward. A goods train does not skid off the starting line like a sports car, but once it has slowly got going, its forward momentum is nonetheless inexorable.

Courage sometimes requires a leap of faith: despite all your planning and preparation, there is still that element of the unknown. When it comes to exercising courage and faith, it is often only once you have jumped that you become aware of the unseen help.

Perseverance

Courage often involves going forward into the unknown or doing something scary. Courage can also involve a more passive endurance of difficult circumstances with patience and fortitude, or it can involve keeping going on a difficult course and not turning back. This latter type of courage is normally called perseverance. An initial fiery enthusiasm is easier than the continuation through fatigue, bad weather or a host of other difficulties.

Perseverance and endurance are, in effect, extensions of courage. It is not failure to experience the temptation to give up, or to wobble on occasions, or to give up, as long as you get going again. Perseverance is normally demonstrated by a continual process of starting again – in other words, refusing to give in to the despair that can arise as a result of initial failure.

For Winston Churchill, there was no such thing as failure, only a learned experience. His motto was: 'Never, never, never, never give up.' When you take that kind of attitude, unseen forces seem to come to your aid. At Dunkirk in 1940, the British Army was defeated. It had literally been driven into the sea. Because of the

range, RAF fighters had difficulty in protecting the beaches and the ships, so the Luftwaffe could bomb and strafe almost at will. The Panzer divisions were only a few miles away – they could easily have wiped the remnants of the British Army off the face of the earth. For no particular reason, however, the Panzers suddenly stopped. The army was gradually shipped back to England in everything from destroyers to river boats. Back in England, it became the core of a new army that would eventually go back to France with its American allies. Once the decision had been made not to give up, everything else somehow seemed to fall into place.

The determination not to give up seems to get powerful forces on your side. Again in 1940, the Royal Air Force was up against overwhelming numbers of German aircraft coming over the Channel to England, bombing British airfields. It seemed only a matter of time before the laws of attrition would work in favour of the Germans. Then something unexpected happened. A German bomber offloaded its bombs on London, the British responded by bombing Berlin, and Hitler went mad and ordered a full-scale bombing of the city of London. The

PERSEVERING

Francis Drake wrote in a prayer:

'O Lord God, when thou givest to they servants to endeavour in any great matter, grant us also to know that it is not the beginning but the continuing of the same until it be thoroughly finished which yieldeth the true glory.'

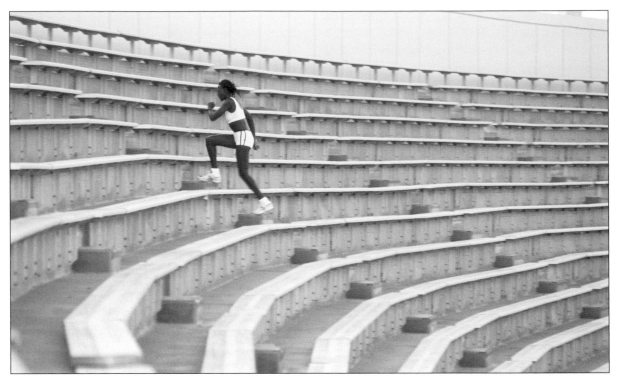

Above: Perseverance means never giving up. Goals are also more likely to be achieved one step at a time, so that the spirit does not become overwhelmed by the challenge.

pressure was off the airfields, and the British were able to continue the fight.

Perseverance is related to persistence, to determination and to endurance. They all defy the end point of failure, which is giving up. The American inventor Thomas Edison said, 'Our greatest weakness lies in giving up. The most certain way to succeed is always to try one more time.' For Edison, there were many 'one more times' until he got it right. When you are on your chin strap, that is the time not to give up. In fact there is only one thing you should give up, and that is giving up itself.

Endurance

Endurance can be both an active and a passive virtue. It means surviving and maintaining the will to go on, despite everything that is thrown at

you. Endurance can mean training all day in the rain, digging a trench and sitting in water all night. It can mean resisting extremes of weather and cold. It can mean continuing with a rigorous training regime day after day, week after week. The difference between the person who endures and those who do not is that he or she climbs out of the mud and carries on.

Endurance involves both physical and mental qualities, though the two are interrelated, and it can be learned. The more the body is hardened and the more the mind is attuned to self-discipline and to the daily round of hard work, the more prepared you will be to endure when the going gets really tough.

At Rorke's Drift in South Africa in 1879, 150 British soldiers defended a supply station against 4000 Zulus. There were several points when they should have given up, but they maintained their discipline and determination in the face of overwhelming odds. The attacking force eventually called it off out of respect for their foes. Endurance had won the day. Sometimes the attacking forces do not relent, but the moral victory remains. The saying 'Remember the Alamo' came about because of the heroism of the defenders of that mission station which, although it was eventually overrun, became a symbol of resistance and the catalyst for Texan independence.

Mind over Matter

The question of whether the mind rules the body or vice versa was discussed by Plato, and has remained a subject of philosophical debate ever since. Plato thought that the two were interrelated and that you could not consider someone's physical health without also considering the health of their mind and soul. Plato was also a dualist, in that he regarded mind and body as distinct entities, with the soul capable of independent existence.

In general there seems to be little doubt that your mind is in charge of your body, but it is also true that the two are interconnected, that they share stimuli from the outside and that each can be trained to perform better. If you have a fit body, it will be much easier for you to carry out a decision to do something such as go out for a run on a cold, misty morning. An unfit body will take a lot more will and determination to get going. On the other hand, if you have allowed your mind to dwell on negative thought patterns, such as anger or resentment or fear, then, even

though your body may be perfectly fit and ready for action, your mind is not able to give clear instructions and directions and the result may be that you miss an opportunity or do not fulfil your potential. The phrase '*mens sana in corpore sano*' (a sound mind in a sound body) relates to this ideal state where we take care of both mind and body so that they function together for optimum performance.

Positive Thinking

Much has been written on the subject of positive thinking and perhaps some concepts in this area have been overcooked. It is not true to say that you can achieve anything you want just by

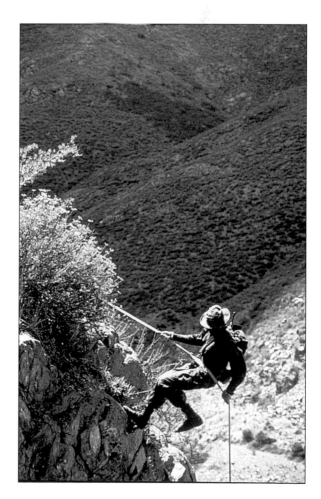

Right: A free spirit allows the mind and body to work together in unison and to achieve optimum results. Here, a Royal Marine commando on a training exercise abseils down a rock face in Wales.

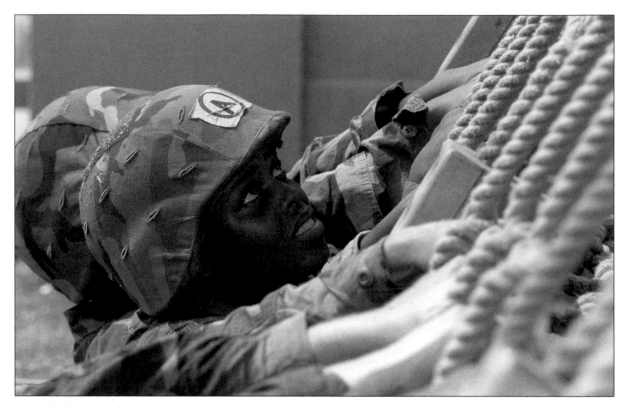

Above: When fear chills the body and the goal seems far away, the refusal to allow negative thoughts to dominate enables you to persevere and to move on.

thinking positively because other factors play a part. It cannot be disputed, however, that positive thinking energizes the body, whereas negative thinking has a dampening effect. Once it becomes a habit, positive thinking can be much easier to sustain, and you can sometimes sense an actual physical reaction when you move from a positive to a negative train of thought. It is as if someone has turned the electricity generator off and power drains from your muscles.

Quite apart from anything else, consistent positive thinking irons out the hesitancy that can make the difference between catching the truck as it pulls away and having to run all the way back to camp. Positive thinking links up to determination and perseverance, and enables

you to hang on in there just a bit longer. For example, a job interview may not have gone too well due to various issues that came up where your profile did not quite match the job. For a negative thinker, these obstacles might be enough to convince him that he might as well throw in the towel, and he leaves the interview room in a resigned state.

The positive thinker, on the other hand, maintains his hope to the last minute. He is still thinking about how this might work out, and when he leaves the room there is something about his eye contact, handshake and remarks that leaves the interviewers with a positive impression and later they are motivated to sit down together to find ways round the difficulties. When they receive his positive follow-up letter the next day, they feel even more inclined to give him a second chance. They do not receive a letter from the other candidate – he was already resigned to failure and that makes the interviewers' decision easier.

When the 27th Armoured Infantry Battalion, Combat Command B, 9th US Armored Division, reached the Ludendorf Bridge across the Rhine at Remagen, on 7 March 1945, there was no time for thinking 'shall we or shan't we'. The bridge had been fully wired up and mined by the Germans, ready for demolition, but without hesitation the Americans rushed it and took the surrounding high ground. In such circumstances, uncertainty or tentativeness might have been disastrous; by not allowing any room for doubt, the mission was successfully accomplished.

Positive thinking in this way tunes the mind and body, and helps it to be ready for any opportunity. Negative thinking or anxiety, on the other hand, can have effects on the body that decrease its efficiency. Peformance, therefore, is related to how we think, and excellent physical performance can only be achieved if the mind is calm and functioning at its optimum level.

The right relation between mind and body is also demonstrated by the ability to practise particular physical movements until they become second nature. This programmes the mind to perform the action without conscious interference. The process can, however, go wrong when the 'programme' seems to short-circuit and the athlete 'forgets' how to perform an action he has performed faultlessly countless

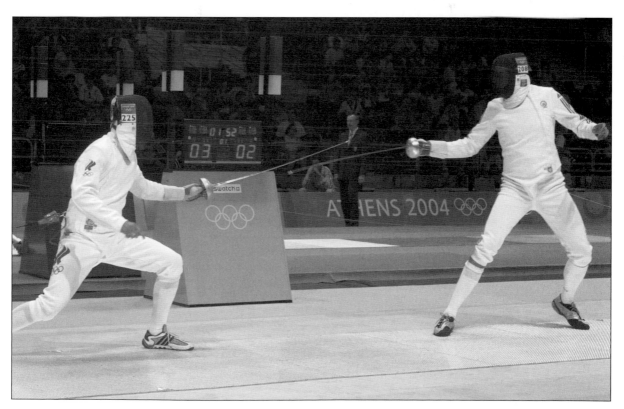

Above: Clear thinking and concentration can produce incisive results when mind and body are attuned. Here, two fencing experts battle it out at the 2004 Olympics in Athens, Greece.

times in training. World-class players have been known not to be able to throw a tennis ball in the air, or to hole an easy putt. This kind of physical freezing is a form of stage fright and results from the tension and anxiety that are a prerequisite of high-level performance.

Although there is no scientific explanation for such problems, it is almost certain that the risk of such performance-related inadequacies can be minimized by positive thinking and visualization. By putting yourself mentally in the frame of what you need to achieve, by visualizing it and imagining yourself overcoming the challenge, you are likely to perform with far greater composure and greater potency. Your positive preparation before the event and your

clear idea about your goal will enable you to overcome all the possible mishaps.

It is no use having ability and training your body to a high level of efficiency if your mind is not up to the job of guiding it in the right direction and keeping it on course. By thinking through potential problems, as opposed to nervously anticipating the worst, you steel your mind to perform on the actual occasion. There could be two problems here, however. One is the unrealistic thought that you cannot do something, and the other is a delusion of grandeur. Both of these extremes may result in the lack of preparation needed for success, as in one case you do not prepare properly because you think you will never make it, and in the other

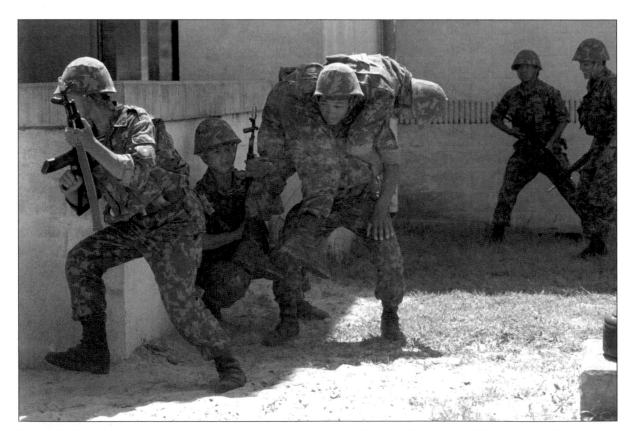

Below: Soldiering is about teamwork and often means carrying each others' burdens. Soldiers have put themselves in extreme danger to rescue their colleagues, as demonstrated in this training exercise.

instance you do not prepare properly because you think it is unnecessary.

Mostly, however, we suffer from a perfectly natural performance anxiety. In this case we tend to think with our emotions, rather than with our mind. That sinking feeling in the stomach becomes the centre of operations, and everything else starts to take its cue from there. We can use patience in these circumstances to still the temptation to anxiety and to maintain rational control of what is going on in the mind. We need to train ourselves not to let our feelings, which are easily swayed by a number of factors, control our decisions and actions. We do what we have decided to do and we do not change our course because of our feelings.

Once you have made a predetermined decision to accept whatever is thrown at you and to make the best of it, everything else will fall into place. It may not be what you decided should happen, but if you accept it as reality at that time you can still use those circumstances to help you move forward. In this way unexpected events, which account for most of the events in the average day, no matter how well we plan, are turned into opportunities as opposed to obstacles. Experienced swimmers know that, when caught in a riptide (the powerful current of water that flows across the face of a beach due to an excess build-up of tidal water), often the best thing to do is not to try to fight the current, but rather to drift and wait until the riptide dissipates, as it eventually will. Having conserved their strength and overcome a sense of panic, these swimmers have a much better chance of swimming back to the shore. Some swimmers drown because they expend all their energy trying to fight the force of the current.

In the face of unexpected events, if we do not use up our energy fighting what is happening and what is out of our control, but instead try to make the most of what is going on and waiting for the next opportunity, we are much more likely to succeed. If, on the other hand, we work ourselves into a frenzy because things have not gone according to plan, we may be in such a state that we fail to notice the opportunities that the new scenario opens for us.

Another problem we come across when things do not turn out the way we had either expected or wanted is that we react with impatience and anger. As you will see from the sections above on patience and anger, these responses can land you in serious trouble very quickly. They can also shield your eyes from the hidden opportunity that lies disguised by unexpected events.

When something negative crops up, another possibility is that you will regard it as inevitable – if your line of thinking is negative. Negative people expect negative things to happen and will interpret difficult circumstances as proof of their theory. Optimists, on the other hand, not only expect good things to happen, but they also make the most of hindrances or are more likely to find a way either over or around them. For an optimist, negative events do not 'make sense', and they keep going until a more positive reality is made manifest.

True Self versus False Self

Thinking something might happen is not necessarily the same as believing it. Some people say over and over again that they can perform some task, but deep down they do not actually believe it. Sometimes a thorough reprogramming of the belief system is required before you can carry through a course of action with conviction.

Some people can be determined enough to perform well on a particular day, but their belief system is too fragile to carry them through.

Military training courses are designed to test how solid you are in this respect. You may be physically capable of taking the pace and mentally tough enough to put up with most of what is thrown at you, but do you have the follow-through and consistent performance that will stand the test of time?

It may well be difficult to distinguish between those who will get through and those who will not. Both people may look the part; both may have equal levels of fitness and intelligence; both may perform to equal standards in training. The difference may be that one of the candidates does not really believe he can make the grade. Somehow the new status he is trying to achieve does not tune in with his inner reality, and this means that at a profound level his confidence is wanting.

Moving into a new role is like an actor learning a part. The difference is that for some that part will become reality, while for others it is always an act. When there is no belief in the part, the danger is that the full force of personality is not fully engaged, and this can adversely affect performance. The other side of the coin is that without putting on the act you never learn the part or gain the new experience. By acting confident or brave we can put ourselves in the way of positive experiences that can indeed help us to build up a genuine store of confidence.

The false self – the personality of pretence rather than the genuine personality – lives on outside experiences and appearances. It models itself on the kind of clothes you wear, the car you drive and the company you keep. There is nothing wrong with this alignment to a certain extent, but it may not necessarily be in tune with your real self, your real values, abilities and limitations. The more you can reconcile your true self with your false self, the more reconciled you will be with yourself and the world, and the more impact you will have. You will also be more likely to achieve your goals. If your two selves are not reconciled, your true self may be constantly

MENTAL IMAGERY

Positive mental imagery is used by top athletes and can also be used by elite soldiers in training. The technique requires practice and refinement, but once it is learned it can be a very useful tool in enhancing performance and overcoming endurance obstacles.

The imagination is a very powerful tool and can be more effective than the force of will. The difference is akin to forcing someone to do something and persuading them. If you persuade someone, rather than force them, they are more likely to deliver.

Start with simple imagery, taking about 10 minutes each day, and go through in your mind the routine of a workout, training session or test. Imagine yourself completing the routine successfully. As you become more accustomed to doing this, you can set your goals higher and start to imagine peak performance. You should imagine as closely as possible the details of the environment you are likely to be in, including the weather and the feel or weight of your equipment. You can also imagine yourself experiencing hunger, thirst, fatigue and the pain of a rucksack pulling on your shoulders, but having the determination to keep going.

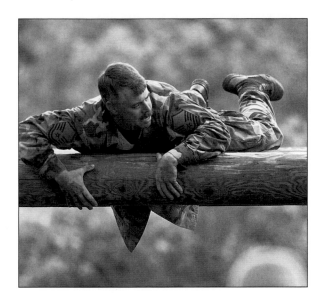

Left: Believing you can has a huge influence on physical performance, and it can mean the difference between success and failure. Military confidence courses are designed to test this balance between mental and physical confidence.

due to you. True success is not about getting your name in the newspapers; it is about using your talents, whatever they are, and developing them to the best of your ability. Success is rated perhaps not by what other people say about you, but rather by what your inner voice says about yourself. Ultimately, you know whether or not you have done yourself justice and, if you feel you have not, do not become discouraged, but have another go.

Self-Doubt

Even highly qualified people go through experiences of self-doubt when faced with taking on a new responsibility or moving into a different job or role. A natural reaction for many people is to think they cannot do it, with the attendant feelings of nervousness. Some people focus on the nerves, and that tends to become a preoccupation. If you learn to accept the unpleasant feeling of nervousness as part of your pre-performance preparation, or as a signal to get your mind into focus for action, then the nervousness can be turned into a positive. It is worth remembering that world-class athletes go through this process, no matter how many times they perform. Once the performance starts, however, it is invariably the case that the unpleasant nerves disappear, drowned out by positive endorphins as they throw themselves into whatever they are doing.

A period of negative anticipation can be detrimental, as some people allow it to influence them too much and therefore convince themselves that they cannot do something. They

nagging at your false self and consequently pulling you down.

One way to reconcile outward and inner reality is to take time to reflect. You may need to allow plenty of time for your true self to absorb the new reality and the new you. If you do this, your true self will begin to adapt and to accept the new reality, and you will move forward with more momentum and impact. Part of this process involves analysing your motives, so that you know you are doing something that is really about you and not about someone else's expectations.

Being yourself involves recognizing your limitations and coming to terms with them. It also means appreciating your assets and making the most of them. By accepting both your assets and your limitations, and accepting who you are, you do not need to be envious of others and you can also let unwarranted criticism bounce off you.

Your particular mix of abilities and personality is unique – no one else has them. By learning to encourage those abilities, developing them and using them in the right environment, you are much more likely to achieve the success that is

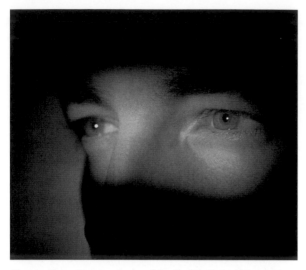

Above: Focus means to banish all else from the mind other than the intended goal. The intense visualization of the goal can often lead to its fulfilment.

difficulties. The second point to note here is that Peter was performing a physically impossible act, but that was secondary to his spiritual and mental engagement. In other words, if your spiritual and mental faculties are properly engaged, you will be able to accomplish what may appear to be impossible.

The third point is that Peter's focus was outside himself – he was not thinking of himself, but focusing on someone else. Obviously this story is about faith, but the point about not focusing too much on ourselves remains valid in any context. We often perform better and feel happier when we are focusing outwards and doing something purposeful.

Fear

Fear can be an emotion that leads us to stop following a crowd and go our own way. It can be a point where, instead of comfortably trying to keep in tune with the expectations of others, we branch out on our own and do something that fits in with our own personality and talents. It takes courage to continue to follow inner convictions, despite what everyone else is saying. Causes of fear are many and various, but one of the greatest is casting out on your own and risking conflict with and even rejection by other people as a result.

Fear occurs in many contexts, such as when you are standing in front of a snarling Doberman, or when you are clinging to a rock face and cannot find a hold. The physical process of fear sends alarm signals throughout your body that it has either to flee or fight, and it tends to close down all systems that are not required for the purpose of getting out of the predicament. Fear is also experienced at the cutting edge, when you know that you are entering an untried area. When considering an action and feeling fear, the trick is not so much to focus on the apprehension,

then fail to take the necessary action because they cannot visualize themselves in that role or because the barrier of negative feeling is too high for them to climb over. By giving in at this point, they deny themselves the benefit of many positive experiences that would enable them to grow and move on.

One way of taking your mind off the negative sensations is to fix your eyes on the goal and to focus on it to such an extent that the other feelings become peripheral and begin to drop away. In the New Testament passage where Peter gets out of the boat and begins to walk across the water towards Jesus, he is fine while he is totally focused on Jesus; however, when his mind begins to focus on the wind and the sea, he becomes afraid and starts to sink.

Peter was doing something most people would rightly consider to be impossible, but such was his focus on his goal, and his faith, that he could actually do it. He had the courage to step out of the boat. The trouble only came when he allowed his mind to focus on the but to reason through what is the worst thing that could happen.

Although there are plenty of reasonable fears, there are also plenty that are unreasonable – known as phobias – and it is worth taking time to distinguish between the two. Try writing down the things you fear. Mark points out of 10 for the likelihood of anything on your list actually happening. Once you have weighed up the evidence, you can then take a truly calculated risk. If you decide that the fear is due to something for which you are not prepared – you may not be fit enough for it, or trained to do it – then make a note to put in the necessary work and preparation before you undertake the task.

We would not survive for very long without fear. It is a self-preservation mechanism to ensure that we think very carefully before taking action that might endanger our lives. Fear produces physical reactions that help us to focus on or to escape from enemies. As with stress, fear is acceptable in small doses, but if it becomes habitual or a compulsion, it will paralyse and also affect health. A large part of fear is 'felt' – in other words, it is generated by the nervous system with proportionate impact on the body. The first thing to realize here is that your mind is in charge of your body, and you therefore have the power to control your fear. Once you have established that your mind is in control and that you do not rationalize with your feelings, you can make a choice either to deal with the challenge or to just move forward, taking the fearful feelings with you.

Nature has equipped the body with the equivalent of a fire service that can drown out the flames of fear and pain. This fire service is made up of endorphins, which produce the feeling of well-being and euphoria experienced when you take physical exercise. If your challenge is physical, you can rely on the unpleasant, fearful, anxious sensations being drowned out once you actually start tackling the challenge. Unfortunately, many of the challenges in the modern world do not involve physical action, but are instead intellectual, political and emotional assaults that leave little scope for dealing with the unpleasant side effects.

If you are being antagonized by someone in a meeting, although you may be physically capable of dealing with that person, the behavioural code does not allow you that option, so you have to learn to cope with the annoyance and spar mentally. The accumulation of anger leads to stress, and this should be vented by regular physical exercise. Fortunately, a

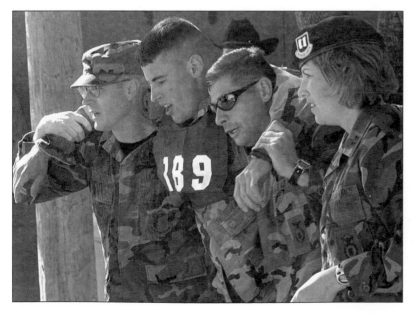

Left: In a team environment, helping your colleagues reach the collective goal is just as important as getting there yourself.

physically fit body is better able to deal with the side effects of mental or emotional stress, and you can get the physical release from the stress of anger through exercise.

Taking Risks

You can possess all the excellent qualities that have been mentioned above – confidence, determination, courage, perseverance and endurance, as well as others – and still not get very far in life. The reason for this is you never actually step outside your comfort zone. You are effectively a Maserati locked up in the garage.

In the story of Peter and the boat, the most remarkable aspect is that he got out of the boat in the first place. It is certainly not the first thing that would come into many people's minds on a stormy night at sea. We are often, however, faced with choices where we either decide to take a leap or come to terms with the fact that it was probably not for us anyway. Or was it? We will never know, as we never tried.

Sometimes we do make mistakes in our decisions, and we have to go back to the fork in the road and try another route. By having taken the plunge, however, we have learned a little more about ourselves and we know we have given it our best shot. By giving it a go, we do not have to live the rest of our lives with that nagging 'what might have been' feeling. Through

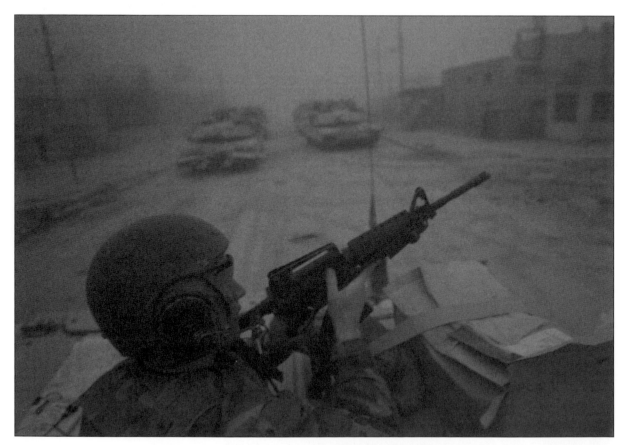

Above: A US soldier keeps lookout on patrol in a sandstorm in Baghdad, 2005. Fear can be overcome, but it also helps us to keep awake and highly attuned in the face of possible danger.

taking risks we grow, even though an enterprise may end in failure. If we can claim to have 'a striving good enough to call a failure', then it is not a failure at all, but rather a stepping stone in our life, part of our story and something that we can look back on in old age with satisfaction.

Not taking risks is a dangerous business, for if we do not take risks we stagnate. The motto of the British Special Air Service is 'Who Dares Wins'. By taking risks, this regiment stays ahead of the game. It is worth looking further at the kind of risks they take. They do not burst into crowded buildings like Wild West gunfighters: they prepare, analyse and train to such a degree that they reduce the risk to its smallest possible size. The SAS has been known to train in mock-ups of the buildings they will assault until every possible move can be predicted. With the risk finely calculated, they go in.

Theodore Roosevelt once wrote:

It is not the critic who counts. Not the man who points out how the strong man stumbled or where the doer of deeds could have done better. The credit belongs to the man who is actually in the arena, whose face is marred by dust and sweat and blood; who strives valiantly; who errs and comes short again and again; who knows the great enthusiasms, the great devotions; who spends himself in a worthy cause. Who, at the best, knows in the end the triumph of high achievement, and who, at the worst, at least fails by daring greatly, so that his place shall never be with those timid souls who know neither victory nor defeat.

One of the biggest obstacles to risk is the fear of failure. People do not take risks because they do not want to be seen to fail in public or they do not want to lower themselves in their own eyes. Perfectionism is the need to get everything

FOCUS

- Clear your mind of everything that is not connected with your goal.
- Reaffirm that your goal is realistic and attainable, and also worthwhile.
- Deal positively with any negative criticism, either from others or in your own thoughts.
- Whenever you have a negative thought, replace it with a positive one which is reassuring and which encourages a 'can-do' attitude.
- Remember your past achievements and how it is that they have brought you to this moment.
- Clear your mind of past and future regrets and apprehensions.
- Concentrate on the particular steps you need to take at this time.
- Give your mind and body time to slow down and rest – practise some meditation.

absolutely right, but perfectionists are often unable to move off the starting blocks.

One way to take risks is the incremental way. Take where you are now as the starting point, and build up each day so that you gradually widen the circumference of your experience and gain new confidence. Rather than throwing yourself into something that you know you cannot do, it is better to overcome your fears by taking a gradual approach and increasing your confidence. Taking risks is about judging the chances of failure and success, then moving forward accordingly. It is not about doing something foolish that you know you are not equipped to accomplish, then proving yourself right in your failure.

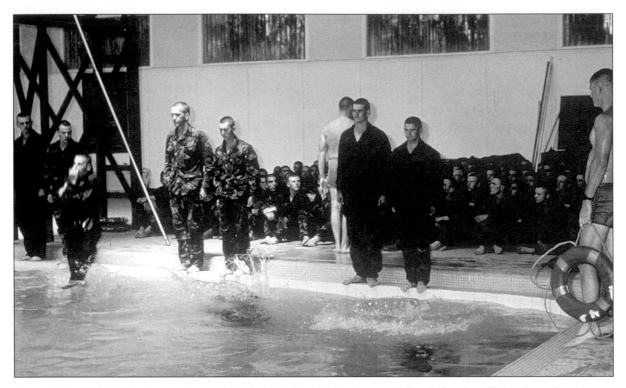

Above: United States Marines undergo swimming training at a boot camp in South Carolina. The trainees have to pass a basic swimming qualification while wearing combat fatiques.

Perhaps the most fundamental aspect of taking a risk is that, although you may put yourself in the way of possible failure, you also stand to win. That is ultimately what risk taking is about – giving yourself the opportunity to grow and to move forward. If you fail, then you have learned something for next time. Perhaps you will be back again when you have had the chance to do a little more preparation.

Frame of Mind

You can read all the above, take it on board and resolve to act on it. The next day, however, you are feeling down. You cannot quite put your finger on it, but you are fed up and you cannot be bothered with changing your attitude. Everything looks grey. If you have spent half an hour stuck in a traffic jam or you have missed the train, thinking positive is not very high on the agenda. Mental discipline, however, does have to override changes of mood that can come about due to a range of outside factors. The essence of mental discipline is consistency, otherwise your performance will be erratic. True mental and physical athletes are people who perform consistently when the going gets tough – they are anything but fairweather soldiers.

Mostly, it is not external events that are the cause of our change of mood, but rather our reaction to them. To learn qualities such as patience, you need to practise them in those circumstances where they are tried, such as getting stuck in a queue. By building up small acts of patience, we are better prepared when something major happens. At some point you have to press the override button and get into the habit of being thankful in all circumstances, as well as spotting the hidden opportunities in each unexpected or apparently inconvenient event. If you get out of bed on a rainy morning and go for a run or a bike ride, you will probably find yourself being thankful for the cooling effect of the rain as your body generates its own heat. You will have conquered the day.

An athlete who has trained him or herself to overlook unpredictable inconveniences is in a much better position than one who has to have everything just right. Elite military forces do not have room for prima donnas. People who suffer from mood swings do not always tend to be bright when things are going well Their negative thoughts can kick in at any moment and make even apparently positive events seem gloomy. As their habit grips them, they become more and more controlled by their emotions and negative mood swings to the point where reason seems to take second place. Furthermore, the more a negative thought is indulged, the more power it gains and the further it gets from reality.

Even where there is a reasonable cause for annoyance, people who indulge negative emotions such as resentment and anger double the power of the original wrong until it is way out of proportion. By harbouring resentment, you in fact do your opponent a favour as you carry around with you destructive emotions that damage your performance and put you in a bad light with other, neutral people.

The best way of dealing with a negative thought or emotion is not to indulge it or to argue with it, but to drop it. The thought can only have force if your mind engages with it, but it will eventually blow away if you refuse to acknowledge it. Instead, try focusing on a positive thought or image. This switch will probably take some effort at first, but will gradually become easier as you replace a bad habit with a good one.

Resentful thoughts are unproductive and are a form of self-indulgence. Often they are a poor excuse for not dealing with a particular difficulty. The more they are indulged, the more harm you do to yourself, so it is better to let them go as soon as possible. Negative thoughts use up your energy as your body responds to the aggressive stimuli signalled by your brain. All that destructive energy is detrimental to your physical health as acids are released into the stomach and as your heart muscle clenches up. Start thinking positive thoughts and you will probably feel an instant change in your body. Energy begins to flow, and your mind becomes more creative. Suddenly, it seems as if the world is full of possibilities.

Cultivating the habit of being thankful for all the events of the day, whether good, bad or indifferent, is a good way of making your mood more positive. Regretting the past is an easy negative thought pattern to fall into. Remind yourself that you cannot change the past, but that you can change the present by doing whatever you are doing well. Some people think that, if only they were somewhere else, such as a sunny country, then everything would be better. This is not always the case, as these people tend to take their moods with them. It is better to change your mood than to change your location.

Another cause of negative moods can be lack of direction and the frustration borne of stagnation. We may have the will to improve our circumstances, but we do not know how. If this is the case, you need to focus on identifying your goals, using professional help if necessary, then setting out to achieve these objectives in a systematic manner. Once you have developed a sense of direction and a goal, you will feel a sense of energy and purpose, and negative thoughts will be brushed aside.

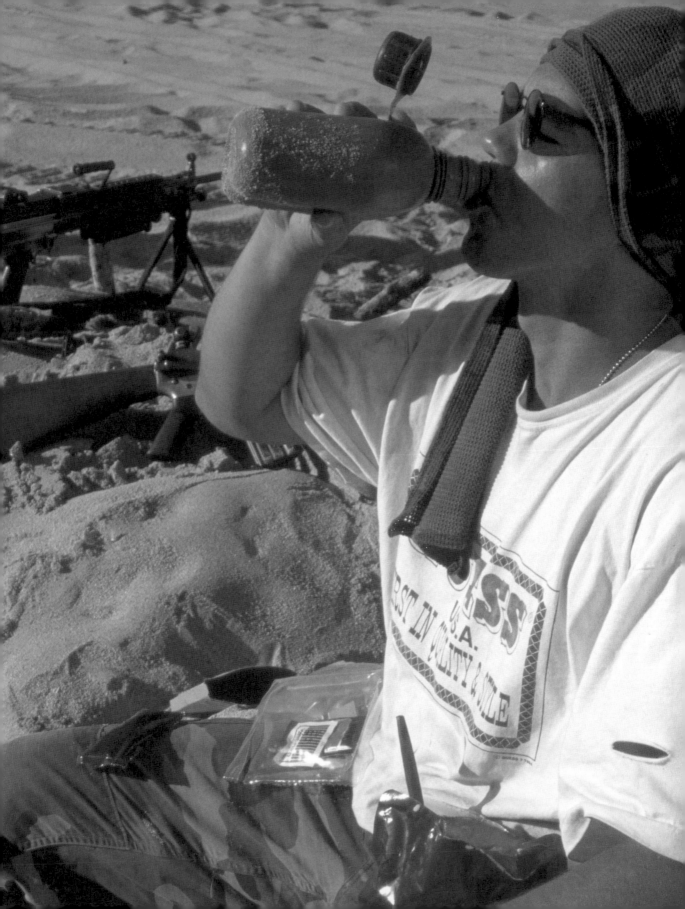

CHAPTER THREE

Diet, Nutrition and Rest

New fuels have been developed for cars that are said to increase performance. Although you pay more at the pump, greater engine efficiency means that you will go further on your gallon of fuel. So, without any change to the vehicle's engine, performance is increased. A similar rule works for the human body.

You may well be at a certain level of fitness, but what you take in to fuel your body will have a significant impact on how that body performs.

Foods can be broadly divided into the following categories:

- Carbohydrates
- Lipids (mainly fats)
- Proteins
- Various micronutrients, including minerals and vitamins.

Each constituent type of food has an effect upon the health and function of our bodies.

Carbohydrates

Carbohydrates are the main source of energy for the body and can be divided into four main groups: monosaccharides, disaccharides, oligosaccharides and polysaccharides.

Monosaccharides are the simple sugars that are found in many fruits and in honey (fructose)

Opposite: Here, A US Marine prepares and eats an MRE (Meal Ready to Eat) in the Saudi Arabian desert, 1999. The correct intake of fluid and food is vital for optimum performance.

and also in yeast and liver (galactose). Disaccharides include sucrose, lactose and maltose. Sucrose is in such things as treacle, syrup and various forms of sugar. Lactose is found in milk, and maltose in malt extract. Trisaccharides are contained in various vegetables, including peas and beans, while polysaccharides include the sugars which are found in cereals.

Fats

Fats are made up of the same elements as carbohydrates – carbon, hydrogen and oxygen – but contain less oxygen. Fats have twice the

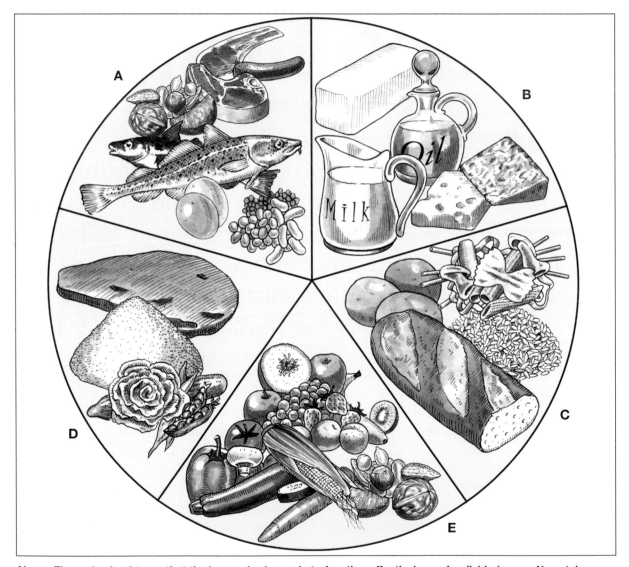

Above: The major food types that the human body needs to function effectively can be divided up as A) protein, consisting of meat, fish, eggs, etc; B) fats and protein from dairy products, such as milk, cheese and butter; C) carbohydrate from bread, cereals and pasta; D) vitamins and minerals from vegetables and meat; and E) vitamins from fruit.

level of kilocalories per equal measure of weight as carbohydrates, and they peform the dual role of providing energy stores and insulator from cold. Fats can be separated into saturated fatty acids and unsaturated fatty acids. The first are normally found in animal fats, while the second are in fish and vegetable oils. Unsaturated fatty acids are known to reduce cholesterol levels, an effect that has a beneficial impact on the health of the heart.

Protein

Proteins are composed of amino acids and contain nitrogen, which differentiates them from carbohydrates and fats. They form a large percentage of muscle (90 per cent), skin (90 per cent) and blood (90 per cent), which is a good indication of their primary importance. They also constitute most of the structure of bones, tendons, hair and nails.

Foods with the highest levels of protein include eggs, beef, milk and fish, as well as oats, rice, flour and maize. These foods are not normally associated with high levels of energy production, but they are vital to the ongoing growth and repair of the body. A report published by the United States Institute of Medicine in September 2002 (*Dietary Reference Intakes for Energy, Carbohydrate, Fiber, Fat, Fatty Acids, Cholesterol, Protein, and Amino Acids*) reaffirms that protein intake for adults should not exceed '0.8 grams per kilogram of body weight'. The report also states that to meet the body's daily nutritional needs, calorie consumption should be split in the following way: 45 to 65 per cent from carbohydrates; 20 to 35 per cent from fat; and 10 to 35 per cent from protein.

A Balanced Diet

Much emphasis has been placed on a balanced diet by nutritionists and government health departments. As no one food can provide all of the necessary nutrients, fibre (essential for digestion) and energy for the body, or satisfy the requirements of body maintenance, growth and repair, a balanced diet is required on a daily basis. A healthy balanced diet should also obviate any requirement for taking vitamin supplements, although this can depend on a

GLUCOSE ENERGY

A system has been developed by nutritionists to measure the capacity of certain foods to increase the concentration of glucose in the blood. Foods with a high glycaemic index include cornflakes, honey, bagels, potatoes, bananas, carrots, white rice, raisins, glucose, sucrose and syrup/treacle. Foods with a moderate glycaemic index include pasta, corn, oatmeal, wholegrain bread, oranges and grapes. Foods with a low glycaemic index include milk, milk products, yoghurt, peas, beans, peanuts, apples, pears, plums, peaches, figs and fructose.

If you consume foods with a high glycaemic index about 30 minutes before taking exercise, you will experience an initial energy rush from the high levels of insulin and glucose, which then rapidly declines. This surge of energy, followed by a rapid drop-off, is not ideal for endurance activities. If, however, you consume foods with a low glycaemic index about 30 minutes prior to taking exercise, the glucose will be absorbed into the body at a relatively slow rate over a longer period – this is an advantage for endurance activities, as it provides a steady release of energy.

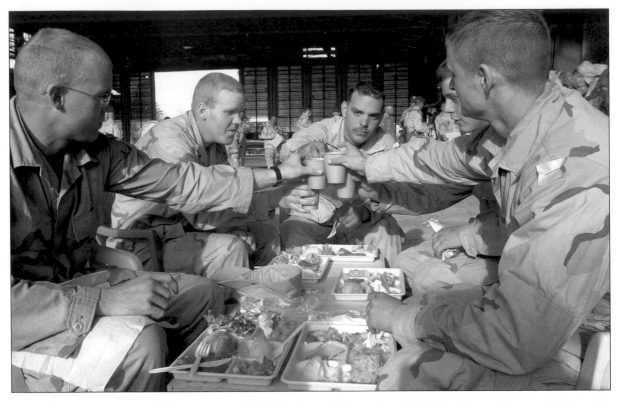

Above: US soldiers at Bagram Air Base in Kabul, Afghanistan, 25 December 2001. Even Army rations can be turned into a decent Christmas lunch with a little imagination.

number of other factors, such as illness, fatigue and stress.

A balanced diet is one which includes a mixture of foods, ranging across the carbohydrate, fat and protein categories and including meat, dairy products, fats and oils, grains and pulses, vegetables and fruit. The 'balance' does not mean that equal amounts should be consumed from all the different categories. For example, there are some foods that have a tendency to increase cholesterol in the body and therefore should be eaten in moderate quantities. The overall aim of the balanced diet is not only to keep a variety of foods in the diet, but also to encourage a large consumption of fruit, vegetables and grains versus a low intake of saturated fats and

moderate intakes of salt and sugar. The bulk of your diet should consist of foods in the bread, cereal, rice and pasta group. Then comes food in the vegetable and fruit group. Next in line are foods such as milk, yoghurt, cheese group, meat, fish, beans, eggs and nuts. Fats, oils and sugars should be kept to a minimum.

Fruit, Vegetables and Grain Products

Fruit, vegetable and grain foods are important as they provide a wide range of vitamins, minerals and complex carbohydrates (starch and dietary fibres), all of which are essential to good health. These foods are also high in calories and preference should be given to gaining calories from such foods as pasta, rice, bread and other cereals, as opposed to meat. Another advantage of fruit, vegetables and grain is that they provide the body with plenty of dietary fibre, which is essential for efficient bowel function and which also reduces the threat of heart disease and other complications.

Fat, Saturated Fat and Cholesterol in Your Diet

Although fat is an essential part of a diet, there has been a tendency in Europe and the United States to eat too much of it. A high level of fat in the diet leads to an increase in the level of cholesterol and a greater danger of heart disease. Lack of exercise, due to increased use of computers and televisions, has tended to exacerbate the negative effect of fat in the diet, leading to obesity. Fat has double the amount of calories per weight than carbohydrates or proteins, so there is every reason for using low-fat options where possible.

Animal fats are made up largely of saturated fatty acids and also contain monounsaturated fatty acids and polyunsaturates. Animal fats are produced as butter, lard, dripping or suet. In addition there are fish oils, though these contain unsaturated fatty acids, as well as the beneficial Omega-3 (n-3) fatty acids and vitamins A and D.

Vegetable oils are derived from oil seeds, such as those from sunflowers or from fruits such as olives. They mainly comprise unsaturated fatty acids and often antioxidants such as vitamin E. Sunflower oil and corn oil contain n-6 fatty acids, while rapeseed and soya oils contain n-3 fatty acids. Olive oil, rapeseed oil and groundnut (peanut) oil are rich in monounsaturated fatty acids.

Fat is a basic nutrient that provides a high level of energy. Saturated fat is also, however, associated with high cholesterol levels and with arterial constriction, and therefore should be taken in moderation. A high intake of saturated fat accompanied by a sedentary lifestyle can put someone in a high-risk category for heart disease. In general, in countries such as the United Kingdom the use of saturated fat has declined, while the use of unsaturated fat has grown. A higher proportion of energy requirements is now taken from wholegrain cereals and from fruits.

Sugar and Salt

Sugars provide instant energy, but foods high in sugar do not necessarily possess much nutritional value. If you have an active training regime, sugars will provide you with some of the energy you need, but they tend to contain excess calories for those who lead a more sedentary lifestyle. In the normal course of events, and with a balanced diet, you do not need to add extra sugar to your diet.

Salt also occurs naturally in foods, and processed foods tend to have salt added. If you add salt to your food, therefore, you are likely to exceed the recommended daily intake of salt or sodium (about 2400mg). A level teaspoon of salt contains about 2300mg. Salt and sodium are also associated with high blood pressure.

Typical Foods from the Different Groups

Cereals

Cereals are a vital source of energy, carbohydrates, proteins and fibre. They are also known to contain a range of vital nutrients such as zinc, magnesium, vitamin E and vitamin B, as well as calcium and iron.

Cereals form the staple diet of populations around the world, and of these rice and wheat are the most important. The use of particular cereals has tended to be proportionate to the type of crops grown in different parts of the world. Rice has therefore been the traditional staple diet in tropical climates, the crop requiring both warmth and plenty of water, while wheat is commonly grown in temperate zones and oats are cultivated in colder climates. The most common use of wheat is in the making of flour. Various breakfast food manufacturers use wheat as the basis of their cereals, which means that this healthy food is often the first item on the daily menu. Maize/corn may be eaten in its natural state, as corn on the cob or as tinned sweetcorn. Maize contains sugars for energy as well as oil. Barley is used to make breads and is high in carbohydrates.

Rice can be eaten in either its brown or white forms. Brown rice has its outer husk removed, but otherwise remains unchanged. White rice is milled to remove the bran and the germ. Rye is used widely in northern countries to produce bread, and rolled oats are found in cereals, particularly porridge.

Fruit and Vegetables

Fruit and vegetables occur in many different forms, for example:

- Soft fruits: raspberry, blackberry, redcurrant
- Citrus fruit: orange, lemon, grapefruit
- Stone fruit: plum, peach, apricot
- Fleshy fruit: apple, pear, banana
- Vine fruit: grape, water melon
- Fruit vegetables: aubergine (eggplant), tomato, cucumber
- Legumes: pea, bean, lentil
- Flower vegetables: broccoli, cauliflower
- Leafy vegetables: spinach, lettuce, cabbage

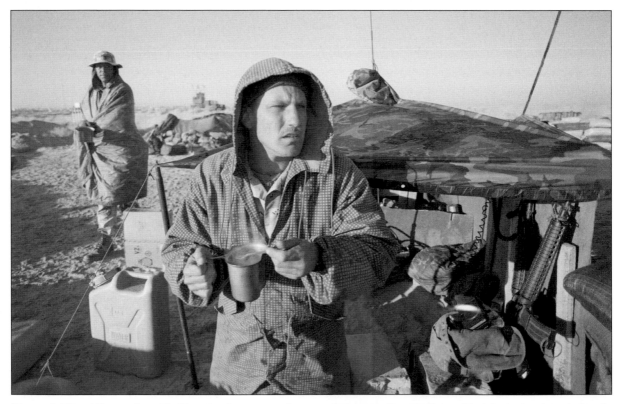

Above: A US soldier stationed in Kuwait takes a warming morning soup after another cold night in the desert. Good diet is essential in extreme weather conditions.

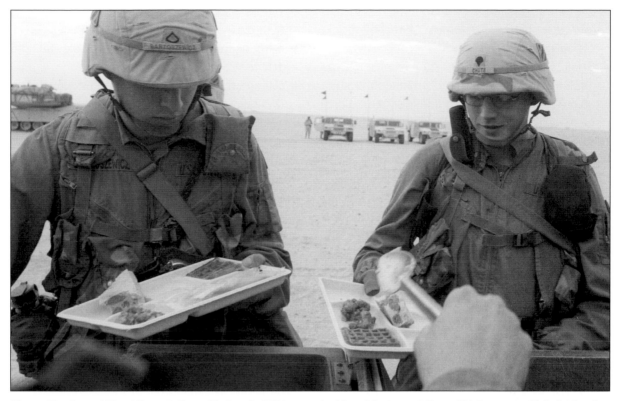

Above: For these US soldiers stationed in Iraq in 2004, a cooked breakfast consisting of high-energy, high-fat foods is the order of a day that is likely to involve considerable energy expenditure.

- Stem vegetables: asparagus, celery
- Fungi: mushroom
- Bulbs: onions, leeks, garlic
- Root vegetables: carrot, parsnip, swede, beetroot (red beet)

Fruit and vegetables are rich sources of vitamin C, beta-carotene and dietary fibre. A diet with a large proportion of fruit and vegetables is thought to reduce the risk of cardiovascular disease and some cancers. Potatoes form a major element of the vegetable diet of European and US peoples. Potatoes come in a range of varieties and are broadly divided between waxy and floury types. They are low in fat and the skin, when eaten, provides fibre. The main part of the potato is a good source of carbohydrates. Potatoes also provide vitamin C, although this can be lost if they are overcooked. The average boiled potato provides about 72 kcal per 100 grams (4oz). The figure tends to be higher when the potatoes are fried, about 189 kcal per 100 grams (4oz).

Fish

Fish's nutritional value is underlined by British government recommendations that at least two portions of fish should be eaten per week, one of which should consist of oily fish.

There are many different types of fish:

- Freshwater fish: for example, freshwater salmon, trout and perch
- Pelagic (swim close to the surface) seawater fish: for example, herring, mackerel and sardine

- Demersal (swim close to the sea bed) seawater fish: for example, cod, haddock, plaice and sole
- Shellfish: for example, molluscs such as cockles and mussels, and crustaceans such as crab, prawns (shrimp) and lobsters.

Fish can also be broadly divided between white and oily varieties. White fish – which include cod, coley, haddock, hake, halibut, monkfish, sea bass, skate, sole and whiting – store their fat reserves in the liver, while oily fish store their fat reserves in both the liver and the flesh. Oily fish include anchovy, carp, eel, herring, kipper, mackerel, salmon, sardine, swordfish, trout and tuna.

Fish is a vital source of protein, providing about about 15–20g (0.5–0.7oz) per 100g (4oz) of meat, and oily fish also provides vitamins A and D. Oily fish contain n-3 fatty acids which are widely thought to contribute to the prevention of heart disease.

Meat

Meat is a good source of protein, as well as vitamins B and D and the minerals iron and zinc. Meat is essentially the muscle tissue of animals and its consistency (tenderness/toughness) tends to depend on which part of the animal it comes from, the age of the animal, its diet and the level of activity of the animal (game tends to be tough). Meat often comes with fat layers attached – these can be cut off to reduce the daily intake of fat.

Milk

Milk is a primary source of calcium, as well as protein, B vitamins and vitamins A and D. It also contains riboflavin, magnesium and potassium. Depending on the type of milk (full cream, semi-skimmed, skimmed) and the amount consumed, milk can also be a major source of fat.

- Whole milk: 3.9g (0.1oz) fat per 100ml (3.5 fluid oz)
- Semi-skimmed milk: 1.7g (0.05oz) fat per 100ml (3.5 fluid oz)
- Skimmed milk: 0.2g (0.007oz) fat per 100ml (3.5 fluid oz)

Yoghurt

Plain (natural) yoghurt is made from coagulated milk that is made sour with lactic acid produced from bacteria such as *Lactobacillus bulgaricus* and *Streptococcus thermophilus*. Bio-yoghurts contain live bacteria.

- Whole-milk yoghurt: about 79 kcal and 3.0g (0.1oz) of fat per 100g (3.5oz)
- Low-fat yoghurt: about 56 kcal and 1.0g (0.03oz) of fat per 100g (3.5oz)
- Greek yoghurt: 115 kcal and 10.2g (0.36oz) of fat per 100g (3.5oz)

Cheese

Cheese is usually made from milk solids or curds that are separated from the milk or whey.

- Cheddar cheese: about 416 kcal and 34.9g (1.22oz) of fat per 100g (3.5oz)
- Half-fat cheddar cheese: about 273kcal and 15.8g (0.55oz) of fat per 100g (3.5oz)
- Edam cheese: about 341 kcal and 26.0g (0.91oz) of fat per 100g (3.5oz)
- Camembert cheese: about 290kcal and 22.7g (0.79oz) of fat per 100g (3.5oz)
- Cottage cheese: about 101 kcal and 4.3g (0.15oz) of fat per 100g (3.5oz)

Cream is made of the separation of fats and solids in milk and butter. Butter is an emulsion of butter fat, water and occasionally salt.

Eggs

Eggs are a rich source of protein and they also contain vitamins A and D, as well as niacin and vitamin B12. When considering the number of

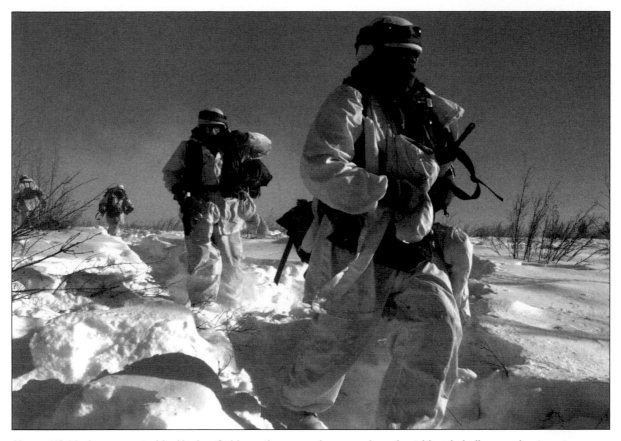

Above: US Marines on patrol in Alaska. Cold weather can raise a number of nutritional challenges due to extra energy expenditure. Exertion in warm clothing can lead to sweating and cold air can absorb body fluid.

eggs that can be eaten, the cholesterol in eggs needs to be taken into account. One egg a day, however, is not likely to raise the cholesterol in the blood. One medium egg contains approximately 86kcals and 6.4g (0.22oz) of fat, of which 1.8g (0.06oz) is saturated fat.

Nuts

Botanical nuts grow on trees and include walnuts and hazelnuts. Legume nuts include probably the most popular and widely eaten nut of all, the peanut. Nuts contain a substantial amount of oil and are rich sources of protein, carbohydrates, minerals and vitamins. They are also high in calcium, folic acid, magnesium, potassium, vitamin E and fibre. Although there is a high level of fat in nuts, the fat content is largely monounsaturated, which has the effect of lowering the cholesterol level in the body. Walnuts contain omega 3 (n-3) fatty acids, which are also beneficial for heart health. Eating nuts is a good way of easing hunger, and for this reason they can be used effectively in some weight-reduction programmes. Some people, however, are allergic to nuts.

Sugar

Sugar is derived from either sugar beet (grown in Europe) or sugar cane (tropical climates). The sugar from these plants is carbohydrate sucrose. The sugars in honey, on the other hand, are mainly glucose and fructose. Sugars of all types provide similar levels of energy, about 394kcal per 100g (3.5oz). Sugars are naturally present in a variety of foods, notably fruits, so some official bodies recommend additional sugar should comprise only 10 per cent of the diet.

Sources of sugar are:
- Granulated sugar: for general use
- Caster (superfine) sugar: fine sugar for baking
- Demerera or raw sugar: large crystals
- Honey
- Golden syrup
- Cane syrup
- Corn syrup
- Maple syrup
- Mollases
- Sorghum
- Treacle
- Soft brown sugar
- Sugar cubes

Chocolate
Chocolate is made from beans of the the obroma cacao tree, which are fermented,

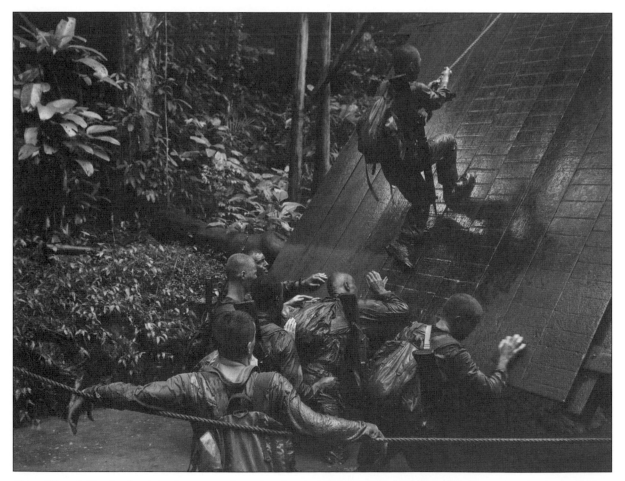

Above: French Foreign Legionnaires sweat it out in a jungle training centre in Guiana. Maximum exertion in the heat can create a critical demand for fluid and energy replacement if dehydration and exhaustion are to be avoided.

roasted and ground. Milk chocolate is made from a mixture of cocoa and milk, while dark or bittersweet chocolate is made without milk. Dark chocolate, in particular, is thought to have significant health benefits, especially with regard to cardiac health, because of the presence of flavonoids, namely epicatechin and gallic acid. These antioxidants help to protect blood vessels and cardiac health, and also reduce the likelihood of cancer.

Chocolate consists mainly of carbohydrate and fat, and a small amount of protein, and contains both calcium and iron. Chocolate also contains a mild stimulant called theobromine, which is a myocardial stimulant with a mood-improving effect. Chocolate tastes good, it is packed with energy, it may improve your mood and it can help your heart. Eaten in moderation, therefore, chocolate is a useful addition to a healthy diet, plus a short-term energy booster.

More Exercise = More Food

If you stand in the food queue at Fort Bragg in the United States or at the Commando Training Centre in Lympstone in southern England, you will not find many people passing over the sizzling sausages and bacon and searching for a salad. Men who will be charging over an assault course, going for an extended run or spending a day on the ranges in the rain need food to power their bodies, especially when they are exposed to the elements, a situation which requires even more energy for body heat. A soldier who eats a fried meal consisting of one slice of fried bread, two sausages, two rashers of bacon, a fried egg, tomato and mushrooms is providing himself with 742kcal, of which 29g (1.02oz) is protein, 57g (2oz) is fat and 31g (1.08oz) is carbohydrate.

The amount of food you eat is relative to your energy expenditure. If there is an imbalance either way, problems may ensue, either in the directions of exhaustion or obesity. The average male civilian needs about 2500kcal per day. The average military recruit needs about 3600kcal per day. Similarly, a male civilian should have a diet consisting of about 50 per cent carbohydrates. A military recruit should have a diet with about 60 per cent carbohydrates. A sprinter might suffer a decrease of muscle glycogen of more than 15 per cent just for running flat out for about six seconds. Imagine how much carbohydrate energy you expend when running a 42km (26.2-mile) marathon, or a 48km (30-mile) route march over the Brecon Beacon mountains in South Wales (a typical challenge for British Special Forces).

If you are faced with a severe endurance challenge, you will need to eat more bulk food such as pasta, potatoes and bread, and you may want to top this off with a slow-release fruit such as dates, or with an energy bar. Note that you will not perform well if you attempt to live almost exclusively on energy foods. If you do this, you will eventually suffer even more fatigue as your body fights to cope with abrupt energy surges followed by rapid energy fall-offs. You need to have a base of slow-release carbohydrate foods (i.e. pasta, bread and so on), and only top it up with the occasional energy booster when necessary. You may want to buy an energy bar, but do not forget that one banana contains 27g (0.95oz) of carbohydrate and provides 105 kcal of energy. A banana is easily absorbed by the body (in other words, your body does not use much energy or water to digest it), and it provides a steady release of energy over the period of exercise. Bananas also contain potassium (beneficial for the heart), vitamin C and fibre. If scientists could have invented a perfect fruit, they would have come up with the banana. You should also remember that you need to replenish energy and depleted glycogen from muscles and liver after you have taken exercise. It is ideal to replace this energy within two hours of the end of the exercise session, as this is the optimum period for rapid absorption.

Military Food

If you are in the military, you will not have much choice over what you eat – you will eat what they provide, unless, of course, you decide to dump your Composite Rations (Compo) or Meals Ready to Eat (MRE) and chase down the nearest rabbit or pluck up the nearest clump of stinging nettles. Unless you are on a survival exercise, however, I would recommend you stay with the military food.

The British Armed Forces 24-hour ration pack is designed to provide one person with a balanced, nutritious diet for one day. It can be eaten either hot or cold, and it provides between 3800 and 4200kcal. The nutritional breakdown in the pack is approximately 55 per cent carbohydrate, 35 per cent fat and 10 per cent protein, and this is broken down into seven menus to cover breakfast, a snack and a main meal, along with drinks (hot and cold). Apart from the standard, temperate-climate pack, there is also a hot-climate pack with extra drinks, a patrol ration pack with more dehydrated food and extra calories, as well as packs which are specific to vegetarian or religious requirements.

The United States forces are supplied with Meals Ready to Eat (MRE), which have gone through a variety of permutations since the early

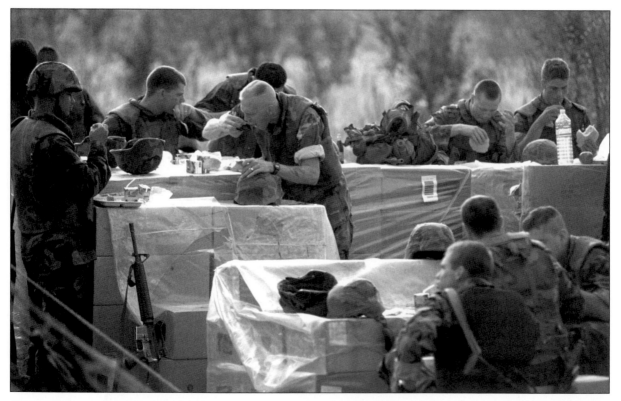

Above: Marines of the 26th Expeditionary Unit refuel on MRE at Camp Monteith in Kosovo, July 1999. The supply of food to forces on the ground is a major logistical challenge.

1980s when alternative unofficial labels included Meals Rejected by Everyone or Many Regurgitated Entrees.

Fluid Intake

Apart from maintaining the correct food intake, you need to take in a substantial amount of fluids if you are to function effectively both mentally and physically and stay alive. If you are exercising in the heat, 3 litres (5 pints) of water per day should be your baseline fluid intake, and you should ideally drink more, depending on the level of exertion and heat.

You do not lose water only in hot climates. Often personnel in extremely cold environments can be in danger of dehydration due to the effects of sweating when exerting themselves in ultra-warm clothing. Most issue rainproof clothing

MEALS READY TO EAT (MRE)

Version MRE XXIV contained the following menu varieties:

- Beefsteak with mushroom gravy
- Pork rib
- Beef ravioli
- Country captain chicken
- Grilled chicken breast
- Chicken with Thai sauce
- Chicken with salsa
- Beef pasty
- Beef stew
- Chilli with macaroni
- Pasta with vegetables and tomato sauce
- Veggie burger with BBQ sauce

- Cheese tortellini
- Manicotti with vegetables
- Beef enchiladas
- Chicken with noodles
- Beef teriyaki
- Cajun rice, beans and sausage
- Roast beef with vegetables
- Spaghetti with meat sauce
- Chicken tetrazzini
- Jambalaya
- Chicken with cavatelli
- Meatloaf with gravy

Menu 4, Country captain chicken, was accompanied by

- Mashed potatoes
- Peanut butter
- Crackers
- Toaster pastry
- Candy (chocolate)

- Hot sauce
- Accessory packet A: coffee, sugar, creamer, salt, chewing gum, matches, toilet tissue, hand cleaner
- A spoon and flameless heater

The edible contents of one MRE should provide abut 1250kcal, broken down into 13 per cent protein, 36 per cent fat, and 51 per cent carbohydrate. They also provide one-third of the Recommended Daily Allowance (RDA) of vitamins and minerals.

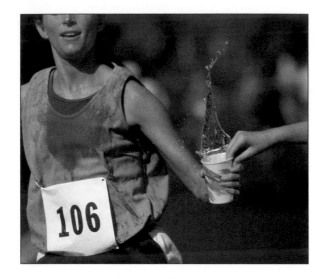

is now breathable, which helps. Any clothing which is not breathable will cause the body to sweat under exertion. You should also be aware of the type of clothing you wear close to your body. For example, inner clothing made from wicking material tends to move moisture out to the outer layers, whereas cotton tends to absorb water and remain damp.

Thirst is not an adequate way to monitor your hydration state. If you feel thirsty, you may already be heading for a serious problem. The best way to monitor the amount of fluid in your body is by watching the colour of your urine. If it is varying shades of yellow, you need to drink water or an isotonic drink. The darker your urine is, the more you need to drink. Little and often is a good rule to follow for fluid intake, but make sure it is not too little.

You should also monitor the amount of liquid in your body by the way you feel. If your head feels a bit tight and slightly muzzy, it may be due to lack of fluids – drink water and your head should feel clearer. If you continue to go without a drink of water, you may get a headache and find it difficult to concentrate. Without water, your brain literally shrinks.

If you drink too much alcohol – for example, on the evening before a run, you will exacerbate the dehydration effect. Alcohol also tends to loosen up the muscles, making them work less efficiently. Coffee and tea can contribute to dehydration because they are diuretic. There should be no problem, however, if you drink a reasonable amount of caffeinated drinks while keeping up a regular water intake. Some people suffer severe withdrawal symptoms from lack of tea or coffee, such as migraines, so if you are planning to reduce your intake of these, it is better to do it gradually over a longer period, rather than drop them suddenly.

Hypotonic and isotonic drinks can be used as a supplement to water, before, during and after exercise. You should learn to judge how much liquid you need to take on board. Too little, and your performance will deteriorate. Too much, and you will need to keep running behind a tree. Make sure that you are stocked up with fluid before any activity such as a squad run where the opportunity to take extra fluid on board may be limited.

Fuel and Exercise Regime

On top of your regular meals, you can top up on carbohydrates before, during and immediately after training. About 30 minutes before you take exercise, you can take on about 25–50g (0.88–1.75oz) of carbohydrates, ideally in the form of a banana, or alternatively a slice of bread with jam, a cereal or fruit bar, or a 400-mil (½-pint) isotonic drink.

If you are exercising for more than an hour, you should consider topping up with between 50 and 60g (1.75 and 2.1oz) of carbohydrates, which could be in the form of dried fruit (about three handfuls), two energy bars, a 100g (3.5oz) chocolate bar or a 1000-mil (1-pint) isotonic drink. When you finish exercise, you should aim to consume 1g (0.03oz) of carbohydrate for every kilogram of your body weight. This will help your body to recover quickly and be ready for the next session. You should back this up with meals made up of complex carbohydrates such as pasta, cereals and bread.

Different environmental conditions can affect your energy output and nutritional requirements. In desert conditions, people tend to reduce their food intake. Because of the loss of water through sweating, fluid intake needs to be kept up and a moderate level of food is needed to replace the salt lost in the sweat. If there is a shortage of water, care should be taken not to eat too much food, as the body absorbs water in the process of digestion.

In cold environments, adequate nutrition is required to maintain energy levels for heat production and to replace energy that may have been lost through shivering. Work in cold environments can be very taxing and uses proportionately more energy. At high altitude, energy expenditure increases due to the reduced oxygen levels and the cold. A higher percentage of energy is used to perform tasks that would be relatively easy at sea level.

Sleep and Rest

There is a tendency to take sleep for granted, but, just as you need more food to cope with an increased exercise regime, you also need to maintain a healthy sleep and rest pattern so that your mind and body can cope with the strain. The fact that somebody is likely to drive a coach and horses through your usual sleep patterns when you are on military training makes no difference to the general rule. Sleep deprivation is part of the testing process of military training programmes, as it is a good way of assessing your underlying character. It also prepares the Special Forces trainee for occasions on active service when normal sleep patterns have to be radically altered. For example, in an observation post or similar scenario, you may run a sleep routine of four hours on, four hours off, which is not particularly pleasant, but enables you to carry out your duties.

In normal circumstances, however, unless you are one of the small percentage of the population who need only three or four hours' sleep per night, you

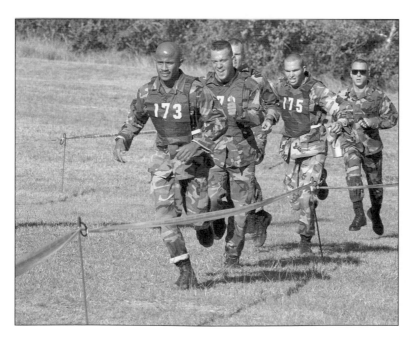

Left: Energy can be boosted and maintained by regular top-ups of carbohydrate, either through energy bars and drinks, or through natural foods such as bananas and dried fruit.

will need to sleep regularly for about seven to eight hours. The good news is that your extra training and healthy living should mean that you are able to sleep soundly.

If you are overtired, however, or worrying about your training programme or about some other problem, your sleep is likely to be disturbed. Negative thinking and depression can affect sleep due to chemical imbalances that cause you to be wide awake at night and yet very lethargic in the morning. You can overcome this by taking care to maintain a positive attitude and by replacing any negative tendencies in your thoughts with positive ones. There is a good and a bad side to most things, and if you get yourself into the habit of looking on the good side you will also train your subconscious to calm down and be more positive.

Look out, also, for other negative signs. Are you seeking powerful distractions of any kind? Do you drink too much alcohol? If so, you may be blotting out something painful in your subconscious. If you cut out the distractions, you may force the underlying problem to the surface. Hopefully the poison or the mental splinter can then be extracted and everything will heal. Sleep sometimes throws up these subconscious worries in the form of dreams, which can be either surreal or straightforward. If you dream about a problem or worry in a straightforward way, it may mean that it has risen out of your subconscious, where it may have been repressed, and that this problem is ready to heal. It may also mark the point where you are now ready to move forward after what may have been a difficult and confusing time.

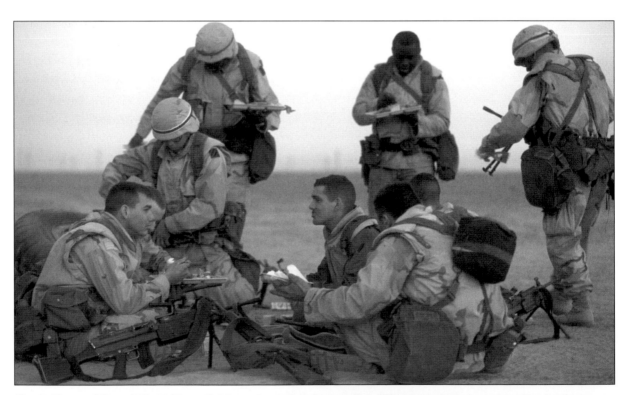

Above: For a soldier, a hot meal is a vital focus for rest and recreation. Efforts are made to make ration packs as varied and interesting as possible.

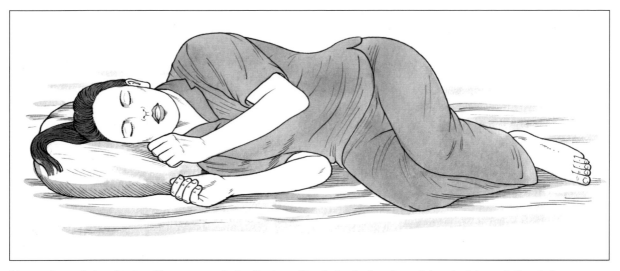

Above: A good sleeping position can maximize the benefits of physical and mental replenishment. Good sleep means optimum endurance and performance when awake.

Lack of sleep will almost invariably affect your ability to concentrate. It may also make your vision hazy or unfocused. It can make you irritable and you will be less able to cope with stress. Lack of sleep causes drivers to crash on roads and is the cause of many fatal accidents. It can cause dangerous incidents in factories and elsewhere. It goes without saying that soldiers, sailors and airmen who handle dangerous weaponry or whose decisions can put other people's lives at risk need to have a grip on their sleeping patterns if they are to perform.

As was demonstrated at the beginning of this book, the crew of *Apollo 13* performed an amazing task in carrying out complex manoeuvres and calculations under extreme stress and while suffering varying forms of sleep deprivation. Yet the idea that if you work late into the night you are somehow achieving more could probably be proved wrong, as, if there is a reasonable interval between work and sleep, sleep itself will probably be more restful and you will wake up more refreshed in the morning. A revitalized body and mind are more efficient than their tired counterparts, and you would probably complete the work you were struggling with at night much more quickly and efficiently the following morning.

Severe sleep deprivation can cause hallucinations, apart from other changes of mood. If your body and mind are deprived of sleep for long enough, you may start to lose control of your ability to stay awake, or your mind will try to sleep while your eyes are open. In hard military training, where sleep is constantly being disrupted, you would need to learn how to make the most of the opportunities that you do get for sleep, which may be in the back of a truck or in a trench, or wrapped up in a sleeping bag under a bush. If you can keep yourself warm and dry, the quality of your sleep may make up to some extent for the lack of quantity. Moreover, if you are being pushed to physical extremes, you should not find it difficult to drop into a deep sleep. Getting enough sleep is a crucial part of your success in training. The better quality sleep you get, the more alert you will be and the better able to cope.

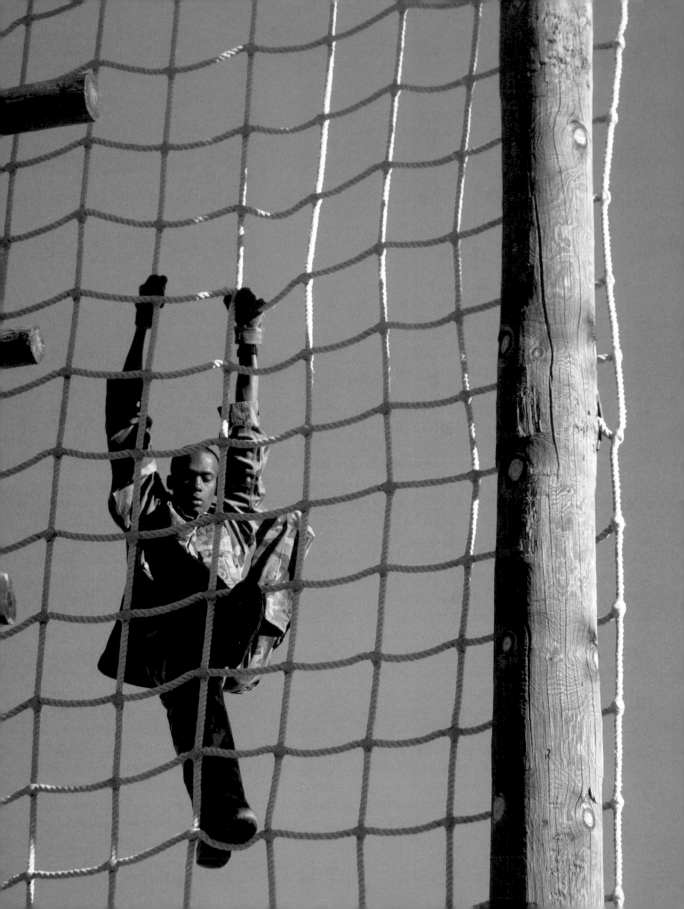

CHAPTER FOUR

Advanced Mental and Physical Training

Now you have achieved a basic level of mental and physical fitness, it is time to learn more advanced techniques that will be directly relevant to live situations and will help you deal with the stresses of combat pressure.

You have been inspired by the stories of endeavour and achievement from the pages of history; you have worked out your goals; you have steeled yourself and brought your determination and commitment up to a level where you can engage in competitive running, swimming, cycling, rowing or even a triathlon.

You have sorted out your attitude and taken a rain check on some of those niggles and relationships that were holding you back. Depending on your initial goal, therefore, whether it was to enter formal military training, to engage in a sport at a higher level, or to set off for an expedition or adventurous training, now

Opposite: A US Army Rangers cadet climbs over an obstacle as part of the intensive assault course open to potential Rangers recruits at Fort A.P. Hill, Virginia.

is the time to pull yourself up to a new and better level of achievement.

This chapter is based on actual requirements of elite forces, and it is therefore recommended that no one should engage in any training which they are not equipped to cope with, both physically and mentally. If your are in any doubt at all, consult a doctor or other appropriate properly qualified professional.

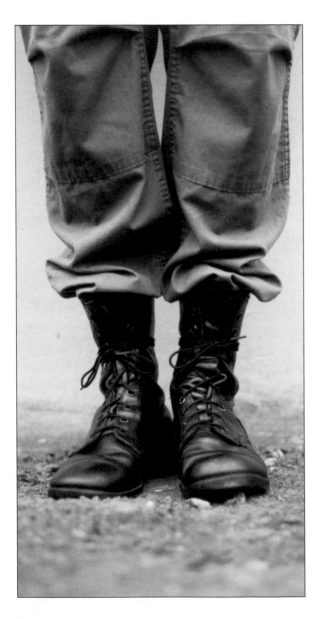

Boots and Bergens

Most of your preparation training will have been done in running trainers or cross trainers, depending on your sport. The human body is not designed to run on tarmac or pavements, and therefore the cushioning from a good running shoe is vital. If you are a tall, heavy runner, you may pronate, which means your foot turns inwards when it hits the ground. This is part of your body's natural suspension system, but if this tendency is too marked it will quickly wear down a pair of trainers designed for neutral runners. It will also affect your running efficiency and may result in injury. You can easily buy shoes with varying degrees of support, most of which will have higher density material on the inside sole of the shoe and/or a plastic block. Some shoe manufacturers have designed their shoes in such a way as to actively steer the foot the other way. The opposite of pronation is supination, whereby your foot tends to tilt outwards. Again, there will be shoes available to cope with this particular tendency.

When buying a running shoe, especially if it is for the first time or a brand with which you are not familiar, it is best to get the advice of a specialist retailer. Do not ask a temporary help in a high-street store or shopping mall, as they may be willing but inexperienced in shoe dynamics. Getting the shoe right will save you time and possibly pain in the future.

When you turn up for training at a military or naval establishment, the sergeant will probably not be very impressed with the note from your mum saying you must always run in trainers because you have delicate feet. You will

Left: Boots issued to US, British and other national forces incorporate running-shoe technology and the latest materials. This greatly reduces the risk of foot, leg and back injuries.

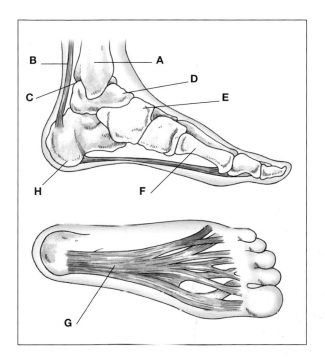

FOOT INJURIES

There are a wide variety of foot injuries, which can result from overuse, falls or poor footwear, including socks and boots. The latest technology utilized in sock systems and waterproof breathable well-cushioned boots reduces the risk of blisters, bunions, Achilles tendonitis and calluses, as well as muscular strains and sprained ankles.

Left: This diagram shows the main bones and muscles of the foot. A. tibia; B. Achilles tendon; C. ankle joint; D. ankle bone; E. talus; F. tarsal bones; G. plantar fascia; and H. calcaneus.

inevitably run in boots. If you find yourself back in trainers, it will be because your feet are not accustomed to boots and you have sustained an injury. You may survive this if you are in regular military training, but not if you are in elite forces training. In short, the sooner you get used to running in boots, the better.

The good news is that boot technology has moved on by leaps and bounds since British forces were suffering trench foot in the Falklands War, wearing hopelessly inadequate ankle boots. The modern-issue boots of United States, British and other armed forces is heaven by comparison. They have soft waterproof leather uppers, well-cushioned soles, excellent support characteristics and are often breathable. They keep your feet dry and well aerated, and help to keep you free from impact injuries.

The dynamics of running in boots are different, however, from running in training shoes. Due to the level of support up the ankle, you will not bend your foot in the same way as you would if you were wearing a running shoe, and the strike on the ground tends to be flatter. You will also often be running in squads, which calls for a regular pace.

Elite forces have a habit of moving over long distances on their feet with all of their equipment on their backs. If you aspire to join them, you need to get used not only to walking long distances in boots, but also to carrying heavy weights on your back. The PLCE bergen currently issued to British Special Forces distributes the weight evenly. The closer the weight is to your back, the less it will pull down on your shoulders. It is also important that the weight should be distributed as evenly as possible between the shoulders and the hips.

When you pack your bergen or rucksack you need to think in terms of the likely priorities when unpacking. In other words, items that you are least likely to need in a hurry should go at the bottom, while items you might need to change into at short notice, such as waterproofs, should go at the top. Each set of items should ideally be packed in a rugged plastic bag to provide waterproof protection, especially if you are likely to be engaged in a river crossing. Other equipment, such as eating utensils, can go in side pockets and/or your belt kit.

Special Air Service Endurance Training

To pass Selection into the British SAS you will be required to complete a number of lengthy walks with weights on your back and carrying a rifle. You will also be expected to navigate accurately and to demonstrate that you are mentally alert at rendezvous points (RVs). The final test is a 64km (40-mile) walk across mountainous terrain carrying a 25kg (55lb) pack, a rifle and belt kit.

KNEE INJURIES

Injuries to the knee tend to vary according to the anatomy of the individual and the kind of activity he or she is engaged in. You can put your knee out by running on uneven ground, but it can also be damaged by bad or worn footwear or footwear that lacks sufficient cushioning. The way your foot hits the ground can affect your knee, and you may need footwear that provides more support against overpronation (where the foot rolls inwards to much) and underpronation (where the foot is rigid and barely rolls at all).

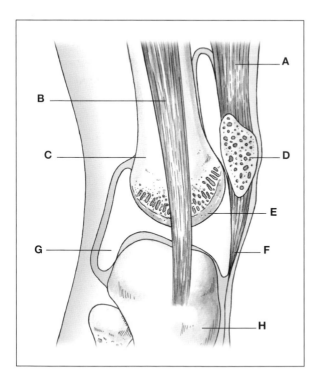

Above: This diagram shows the main bones and muslces of the knee. A. tendon of quadriceps muscle, B. Iliotibial band, C. femur, D. patella, E. cartilage, F. patella ligament, G. synovial membrane, H. tibia.

To attain anything like the required level of fitness, you will need to work up your carrying capacity and the distance you walk in achievable stages. You can start off with as little as 15kg (33lb) in your backpack and walk for about 13km (8 miles). Increase your next walk to about 19km (12 miles), raising the weight in your pack to about 18kg (40lb). If you are serious about passing Selection, you will need to keep your eye on your watch: you will want to cover 20km (12½ miles) in less than four hours. You may continue gradually to increase the weight in your backpack until you have reached about 25kg (55lb). At this stage you may feel fit enough to attempt a 40km (25-mile) hike.

A good place to practise this sort of walking is in hilly country. The walk up to Pen y Fan in the Brecon Beacons (a mountainous area of South Wales, UK, used by the SAS in training) provides a good test of endurance, especially in view of the many false horizons you encounter as you ascend. It will test both your physical endurance and your mental determination.

British Royal Marine Commando Training

In the Royal Marines, before going on for further training and the Commando Course itself, you will first need to able to successfully complete the following Basic Fitness Test:

1. Upper body exercises consisting of five pull-ups and 50 sit-ups.
2. A squad run and walk of 2km (1¼ miles) in 15 minutes.
3. A run over 2km (1¼) miles in less than 12 minutes.

The official procedure for completing the pull-ups and sit-ups is as follows:

Pull-ups

a. Hang from the bar with a hand-over grip, your hands shoulder-width apart, and arms and body straight.
b. Bend your arms until your chest is up to the level of the bar and your chin is over the bar. Keep your body straight at all times, including the legs.

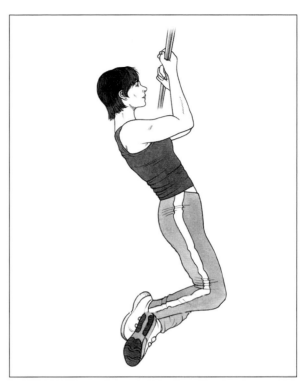

Above: To perform pull-ups, hang from a horizontal bar, with knees bent if necessary to keep your feet off the ground. Pull yourself up until your chin is over the bar. Lower your body to the original hanging position and repeat. The aim is to maintain control throughout.

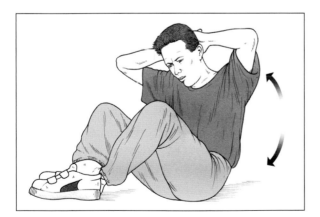

Above: To do crunches, lie on your back with knees bent and feet flat on the floor. Place your hands behind your head. Raise your upper body as far as you can, then lower it under control. Repeat.

c. Lower your body to the starting position, until both arms and body are completely straight again. Repeat.

Sit-ups

Lie on the ground or on a mat with knees bent, feet flat on the ground and no more than 8cm (3in) apart. Bend the arms, with elbows pulled back, fingertips on the temples. A partner must hold down your feet for the exercise.

a. Bring the upper body up to the vertical, while keeping the hips on the floor and fingers on the temples.
b. Return to the starting position, making sure that both shoulder blades and the back of the

head make contact with the ground before repeating the sit-up.

c. Perform sit-ups for two minutes or until candidate can no longer continue. Rest periods are allowed, without changing essential position.

The Basic Fitness Test is followed by Basic Training. This challenges all-round body strength for carrying weights, and upper-body strength tests include climbing ropes while wearing 15kg (32lb) of equipment, a battle swimming test and a 'regain' – climbing back up a rope suspended over a water tank. The Commando Course itself includes climbing and ropework techniques, patrolling and various amphibious operations.

Typical challenges include:

- 10km (6-mile) speed march in full fighting order to be completed in 60 minutes.
- Endurance course: tunnels, pipes, wading pools and an underwater culvert; 10km (6-mile) run back to base; marksmanship test; completion time 72 minutes for men, 70 minutes for officers.
- Tarzan assault course: assault course combined with aerial confidence course; includes death slide and rope climb up 9m (30ft) wall; to be completed in full fighting order in 13 minutes, 12 minutes for officers.
- 15km (9-mile) speed march: recruits required to complete speed march in 90 minutes carrying full fighting order.

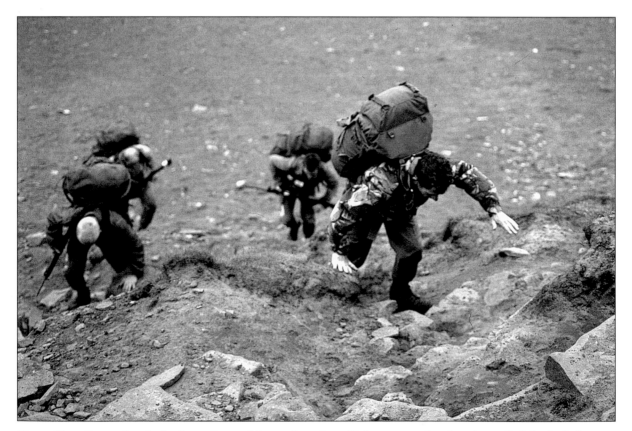

Above: Recruits require plenty of practice walking and running with bergens and rucksacks on their backs before attempting arduous elite selection courses such as SAS Selection.

● 48km (30-mile) march across Dartmoor (in Devon) wearing full fighting order and additional safety equipment. This must be completed in eight hours for recruits and seven hours for officers. Officers are responsible for their own navigation, while recruits march as a syndicate with navigation carried out by a member of the directing staff (DS).

Retakes for any failed tests take place the day after the final test.

On successful completion of the Commando Course, Royal Marines go on to specialist training, which may include a mountain leader course (skiing and Arctic warfare), amphibious training, sniper training and PT instructor.

British Parachute Regiment Selection – 'P' Company

'P' Company lasts for one week and includes the following sequential elements:

1. The Steeplechase: this is a 3km (2-mile) course with 25 obstacles that must be completed in 19 minutes. It tests overall cardiovascular fitness.
2. The Trainasium: this aerial apparatus tests aptitude for training at heights, as well as individual courage.
3. The Log Race: a team race carrying a heavy log round a 3km (2-mile) course. Everybody has to keep up with everybody else and it can be a killer if you are taller than the rest, which means either you carry most of the weight or you have to bend down and run in a crouch!
4. Stretcher Race: a team race with each group of soldiers carrying a weighted stretcher. This again tests team cohesion, and you will feel like you need a stretcher at the end of it.
5. Milling: a one-minute boxing bout that is designed as a test of your aggression. Ideally, you do not want the other guy to be seen to be taking all the initiative.

6. 16km (10-mile) march: you will carry a 16kg (35lb) bergen and a weapon, and you will be expected to complete the 16km (10 miles) in one hour and 50 minutes.
7. 32km (20-mile) endurance march: you will carry a 16kg (35lb) bergen and a weapon, and you will be expected to complete the march in five hours.

Navy SEALS Preparation Workout

The Navy SEALs also issue a suggested preparation workout, schedule II.

These workouts have been designed to produce muscle endurance. As you move on with the workouts, it should take longer for your

Actual Requirements for Selection by the United States Navy Sea Air Land (SEAL) Forces

PHASE	
1	Pass or fail on the following: • 50m (164ft) underwater swim • Underwater knot tying • Drown-proofing test • Basic lifesaving test
	Timed tests: • 1200m (336ft) pool swim with fins – 45 min • 1.6km (1-mile) bay swim with fins – 50 min • 1.6km (1-mile) ocean swim with fins – 50 min • 2km (1¼-mile) ocean swim with fins – 70 min • 3km (2-mile) ocean swim with fins – 95 min • Obstacle course – 15 min • 6km (4-mile) timed run – 32 min
	Timed/conditioning tests • 2000m (6561ft) conditioning pool swim without fins – to completion • 2km (1?-mile) night bay swim with fins – to completion • 3km (2-mile) ocean swim with fins – 85 minutes • 6km (4-mile) timed run – 32 minutes • Obstacle course – 13 minutes
2	• 3km (2-mile) ocean swim with fins – 80 min • 6km (4-mile) timed run in boots – 31 min • Obstacle course – 10:30 completion time. • 6km (3¾-mile) ocean swim with fins – to completion • 9km (5½-mile) ocean swim with fins – to completion
3	• Obstacle course – 10 min • 6km (4-mile) timed run in boots – 30 min • 23km (14-mile) run – to completion • 3km (2-mile) ocean swim with fins – 75 min

United States Navy SEALs Suggested Running Training Schedule II

WEEK	
1	Mon: 5km (3 miles) Tues: 8km (5 miles) Thurs: 6km (4 miles) Fri: 8km (5 miles) Sat: 3km (2 miles) Total: 30km (19 miles)
2	Mon: 5km (3 miles) Tues: 8km (5 miles) Thurs: 6km (4 miles) Fri: 8km (5 miles) Sat: 3km (2 miles) Total: 30km (19 miles)
3	Mon: 6km (4 miles) Tues: 8km (5 miles) Thurs: 10km (6 miles) Fri: 6km (4 miles) Sat: 5km (3 miles) Total: 35km (22 miles)
4	Mon: 6km (4 miles) Tues: 8km (5 miles) Thurs: 10km (6 miles) Fri: 6km (4 miles) Sat: 5km (3 miles) Total: 35km (22 miles)
5	Mon: 8km (5 miles) Tues: 8km (5 miles) Thurs: 10km (6 miles) Fri: 6km (4 miles) Sat: 6km (4 miles) Total: 38km (24 miles)
6	Mon: 8km (5 miles) Tues: 10km (6 miles) Thurs: 10km (6 miles) Fri: 10km (6 miles) Sat: 6km (4 miles) Total: 44km (27 miles)
7	Mon: 10km (6 miles) Tues: 10km (6 miles) Thurs: 10km (6 miles) Fri: 10km (6 miles) Sat: 10km (6 miles) Total: 50km (30 miles)

United States Navy SEALs Physical Training Schedule II (Mon/Wed/Fri)

WEEK	
1	6 x 3 push-ups 6 x 5 sit-ups 3 x 10 pull-ups 3 x 20 dips
2	Ditto
3	10 x 20 push-ups 10 x 25 sit-ups 4 x 10 pull-ups 10 x 15 dips
4	Ditto
5	15 x 20 push-ups 15 x 25 sit-ups 4 x 12 pull-ups 15 x 15 dips
6	20 x 20 push-ups 20 x 25 sit-ups 5 x 12 pull-ups 20 x 15 dips

Pyramid Workouts

The object of a pyramid workout is to work up to a set goal, for example five, then gradually work down again to where you started.

Number of repetitions:
Pull-ups: 1, 2, 3, 4, 5, 4, 3, 2, 1
Push-ups: 2, 4, 6, 8, 10, 8, 6, 4, 2 (in other words, twice the number of pull-ups)
Sit-ups: 3, 6, 9, 12, 15, 12, 9, 6, 3 (in other words, three times the number of pull-ups)
Dips: 1, 2, 3, 4, 5, 4, 3, 2, 1

To avoid strain and injury to foot muscles, the SEALs recommend that the recruit swims 1000m (3280ft) with fins and 1000m (3280ft) without. The speed goal should be to swim 50m (164ft) in 45 seconds or less.

muscles to tire. Try to alternate sets of exercises so that one set of muscles has a chance to rest while the other works.

Once you have graduated from schedule II, you can move on to the more varied pyramid workouts.

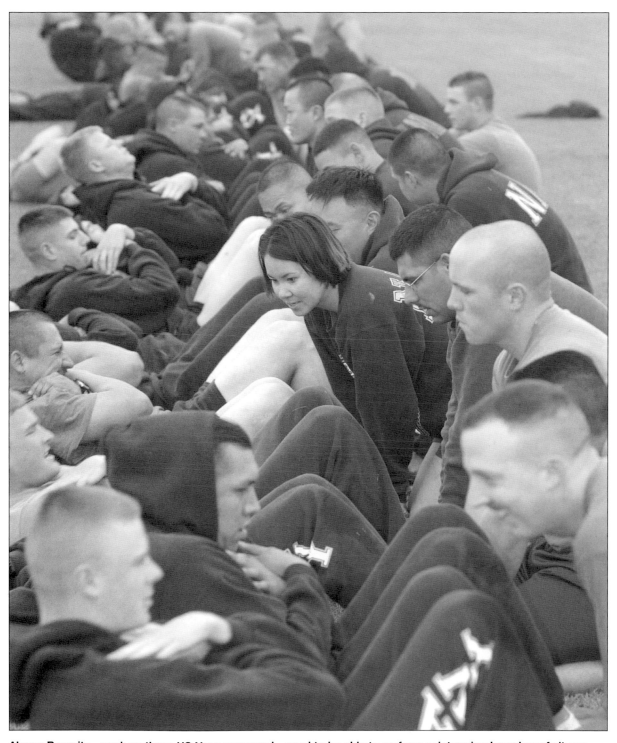

Above: Recruits – such as these US Navy personnel – need to be able to perform a determined number of sit-ups to pass through basic selection for certain military courses.

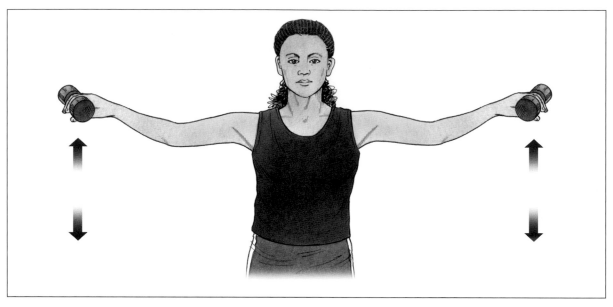

Above: To perform side lateral raises, standing straight with your feet evenly spaced and the barbells by your side, raise the barbells to shoulder level, then down again. Repeat.

Stretching

While Monday, Wednesday and Friday are devoted to physical training, Tuesday, Thursday and Friday can be devoted to stretching. The US Navy SEALs recommend a 15-minute stretch before any workout, with the emphasis placed on the muscles used in the last workout. Start at the top of the body and work down, taking care not to bounce on the stretch and holding the stretch for 10–15 seconds. They also recommend concentrating particularly on thighs, hamstrings, chest, back and shoulders.

United States Marine Corps – Combat Water Survival/Qualification Standards and Test Procedures

Many of the elite forces training programmes contain an element of water training and testing, with an obvious emphasis in the marines and other waterborne Special Forces (Special

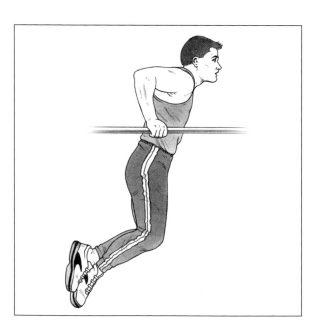

Right: To perform parallel bar dips, stand between the parallel bars, holding them with each hand, and lift your body off the ground until your arms lock. Cross your legs and bend your knees, then lower your body until your upper arms are parallel with the bars. Repeat 10 times or until tired.

Forces). The programme below is the test standards for the US Marines in various grades.

According to the manual, the tests are carried out 'while wearing full combat gear unless otherwise stated. Full combat gear will consist of boots, utilities, helmet, flack jacket, H-harness, cartridge belt, two magazine pouches, two full canteens with covers, rubber rifle, and a standard 40-pound pack, with frame, which has been properly waterproofed. Gas mask, first-aid kit, magazines, sopor mats, and sleeping bags will not be used during testing or training.'

Swimming Workout II (4 or 5 days per week)

WEEK	
1	Swim continuously for 35 minutes
2	Swim continuously for 35 minutes
3	Swim continuously for 45 minutes with fins
4	Swim continuously for 45 minutes with fins
5	Swim continuously for 60 minutes with fins
6	Swim continuously for 75 minutes with fins

Combat Water Survival, Third Class (CWS3)

- Enter shallow water (minimum 1m/3ft) with weapon and wearing full combat gear.
- Walk 20m (66ft) in shallow water (minimum 1m/3ft waist deep) with weapon at port arms and wearing full combat gear.
- Walk 40m (131ft) in chest-deep water wearing full gear and weapon (weapon slung around neck) using a modified breaststroke arm movement and modified combat stroke leg movement (bicycle stroke).

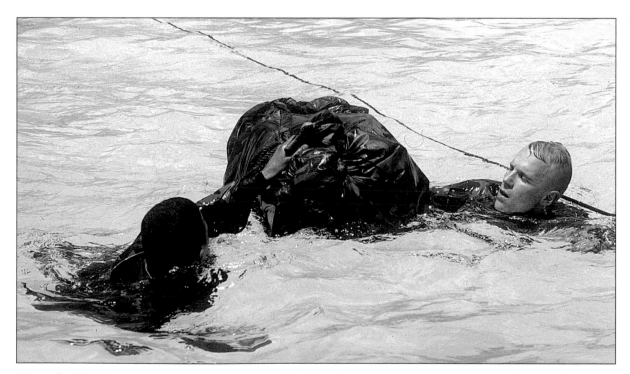

Above: Combat water survival training is a prerequisite for marines and other waterborne special forces. Other elite units also train regularly to cross rivers and other water obstacles safely with all their equipment.

- Travel for 40m (131ft) in deep water (over the head) with full gear and weapon.
- Enter water from height of 1.5m (5ft) using the modified abandon ship technique, into deep water with full gear and weapon (weapon inverted at sling arms), travel 10m (32ft), remove pack, and travel 15m (49ft) with pack and weapon.
- Jump from minimum height of 2.4m (8ft), maximum of 4.6m (15ft), using the abandon ship technique wearing utilities and boots only and travel 25m (82ft) using either a beginner swimming stroke (on front or back) or demonstrating a basic knowledge of any survival stroke or combination thereof.

Combat Water Survival, Second Class (CWS2)

Develop skill level to be able to assist a wounded Marine to safety. Must have completed CWS3. Uniform will be full combat gear and contents of pack will be waterproofed.

- With full combat gear minus pack, swim 50m (164ft) in deep water, with weapon slung across back (muzzle down).
- Wearing full combat gear, perform 25m (82ft) collar-tow on passive 'victim' similarly dressed, simultaneously towing two packs and two weapons (secured to packs). Packs may be used for floatation devices for 'victim'.

Combat Water Survival, First Class (CWS1)

- Demonstrate ability to rescue yourself, assist a distressed swimmer to safety, and survive under adverse situations. Must have completed CWS2. Steps will be executed in sequence wearing only the utility uniform (no boots).
- Survival strokes: Properly demonstrate the following:
  25m (82ft) breaststroke
  25m (82ft) sidestroke
  25m (82ft) elementary backstroke

Opposite: Canoe rolling is about maintaining momentum so that the body and canoe continue to move throughout the roll. The rear of the paddle is sliced into the water, minimizing resistance. The canoeist crouches forwards and waits for the right moment before sweeping back with the blade to complete the roll and bring him or herself upright.

- Rescues: dry land drill, water demonstration, and student practice time of all three rescues. Students must properly demonstrate each rescue for qualification, utilizing ease-in entry technique with victim 5m (16ft) away. Victims are passive during carry or tow.
- Front head hold escape, front surface approach, wrist tow for 25m (82ft).
- Rear head hold escape, rear approach, double armpit tow, cross-chest carry for 25m (82ft).
- Double wrist grip escape, swimming assist to the front.
- Swim 250m (820ft) using one or a combination of survival strokes.

Water Survival Qualified (WSQ)

Successful completion of CWS1 and the following procedures are prerequisites for WSQ.

- Splash Recover Technique. Swim underwater 10m (32ft), on the surface 40m (131ft) in simulated burning oil spill situation. Uniform will be utilities and boots.
- Abandon ship technique; enter water from a height greater than 2.4m (8ft) but less than 4.5m (15ft).
- Without surfacing, swim 10m (32ft).
- Using splash technique, go to surface.
- Remain on surface, use modified breaststroke splashing technique, and swim 40m (131ft).
- Enter water in full combat gear from a minimum height of 2.4m (8ft) – max 49ft (15ft) – using abandon ship technique.

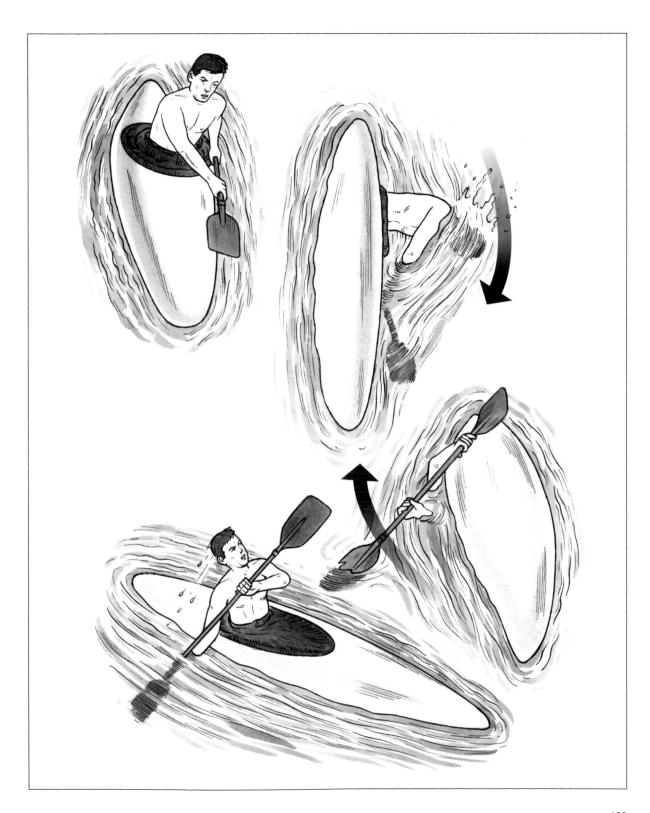

ADVANCED MENTAL AND PHYSICAL TRAINING

- Remove pack, assume a reconnaissance position utilizing the pack, traverse 25m (82ft) simulating sighting in and engaging enemy on either flank.
- Tread water or survival float in deep water

with utilities and boots for 30 minutes without artificial flotation. Boots will be removed after five minutes and retained. Five minutes prior to completion of the 30-minute float, and without exiting from the water, replace the

Suggested Workout Based on Preparation for US Ranger School

WEEK	MON	TUES	WED	THUR	FRI	SAT	SUN
1	Hard: 100m (328ft) swim nonstop, without touching sides or bottom of pool. Forced march with rucksack (quarter of your body weight): 5km (3 miles) in 60 minutes cross country.	Easy: Stationary bike or real bike ride: 20 minutes at 70 per cent heart rate. Skipping 10 minutes.	Hard: 3 sets (maximum repetitions) of push-ups in 30 seconds. 5km (3-mile) run (moderate pace) Rope climb or 3 sets of maximum repetitions chin-ups. Forced march with rucksack (quarter of your body weight): 8km (5 miles) in 1 hour 40 minutes cross country.	Easy: Stationary bike or real bike ride: 20 minutes at 70 per cent heart rate. 40m (64ft) sprints (10 times with 30 seconds rest) 15m (49ft) swim in full uniform and boots	Hard: Forced march with rucksack (quarter of your body weight): 8km (5 miles) in 1 hour 40 minutes cross country	Easy: 3 sets of push-ups and sit-ups (maximum repetitions in 30 seconds) 3 sets of chin-ups (maximum repetitions) 200m (656ft) swim	REST
2	Hard: Forced march with rucksack (? of body weight): 13km (8 miles) in 2 hours and 40 minutes cross country	Easy: Stationary bike or real bike ride: 20 minutes at 70 per cent heart rate	Hard: 3 sets (maximum repetitions) of push-ups, chin-ups and sit-ups in a 35-second period. 8km (5-mile) run (moderate pace) 3 sets (30–50 each) of squats with rucksack (quarter body weight). Drop down to 90-degree angle between upper and lower leg	Easy: 300m (984ft) swim nonstop. Any stroke, apart from backstroke	Hard: Forced march with rucksack (quarter body weight); 16km (10 miles) in 4 hours cross country	Easy: 3 sets (maximum repetitions) of push-ups, chin-ups, and sit-ups in a 35-second period Stationary bike or real bike ride: 20 minutes at 80 per cent heart rate. 15m (49ft) swim in full uniform (BDU) and boots	REST
3	Hard: 4 sets of maximum push-ups, chin-ups, and sit-ups in a 40-second period. 6km (4-mile) run (fast to moderate pace) 4 sets (50 each) of squats with rucksack (quarter body weight). Drop down to 90-degree angle between upper and lower leg	Easy: Stationary bike or real bike ride: 20 minutes at 20 per cent heart rate. Skip for 12 minutes	Hard: Forced march: 19km (12 miles) with rucksack (quarter body weight or 27kg/60lb, whichever is greater) in 3 hours along road or 4 hours cross country.	Easy: Swim 400m (1312ft)	Hard: 4 sets (maximum repetitions) of push-ups, chin-ups, and sit-ups in a 40-second period. 10km (6-mile) run (fast to moderate pace)	Easy: Stationary bike or real bike ride: 20 minutes at 80 per cent heart rate Skipping 10 minutes nonstop 15m (49ft) swim in full uniform (BDUs) and boots	REST

Suggested Workout Based on Preparation for US Ranger School

WEEK	MON	TUES	WED	THUR	FRI	SAT	SUN
4	Hard: Forced march 13km (8 miles) with rucksack (quarter body weight or 27kg/60lb, whichever is greater) in 2 hours along road or 2 hours 40 minutes cross country	Easy: Swim 400m (1312ft) 4 sets of dips, push-ups, chin-ups and sit-ups in a 40-second period.	Hard: 10km (6-mile) run (fast to moderate pace) 3 sets (12 repetitions) leg presses, heel raises, leg extensions, leg curls	Easy: 4 sets push-ups, chin-ups, and sit-ups in a 40-second period (maximum repetitions) Stationary bike or real bike ride: 25 minutes at 80 per cent maximum heart rate.	Hard: Forced march: 19km (12 miles) with rucksack (quarter body weight or 34kg/75lb, whichever is greater) in 4 hours cross country	Easy: 4 sets push-ups, chin-ups, and sit-ups in a 40-second period (maximum repetitions) 15 minutes skipping.	REST
5	Hard: 5km (3-mile) run (fast pace). 500m (1640ft) swim (nonstop, any stroke other than backstroke) 3 sets (8–12 repetitions) of leg presses, heel raises, leg extensions, leg curls	Easy: Skipping 12 minutes nonstop	Hard: Army Personal Fitness Test	Easy: Swim 400m (1312ft) 4 sets dips (maximum repetitions)	Hard: Forced march 29km (18 miles) with rucksack (quarter body weight or 34kg/75lb, whichever is greater) in 4 hours 30 minutes along road or 6 hours cross country	Easy: 4 sets push-ups, chin-ups, and sit-ups in a 40-second period (maximum repetitions) Skipping 12 minutes nonstop	REST

boots and swim 500m (1640ft) using one or a combination of survival strokes.

● Trouser inflation/back float for 1 minute.

Advanced Mental Endurance

Having achieved a high level of fitness will certainly help your self-confidence; however, although you may be physically capable of taking the pace, the key to success is your mental endurance – your ability not only to keep going, but also to maintain a calm attitude despite everything that is thrown at you and to continue to operate efficiently and successfully in rigorous conditions.

A Special Forces soldier needs to be ahead of the game at all times, using his initiative and always being thoroughly aware. Special Forces soldiers need to be able to operate on their own,

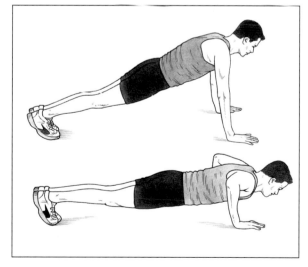

Above: When doing press-ups, place your hands flat on the ground, shoulder-width apart. Keep your back straight at all times and bend with your arms, so that all the pressure is concentrated in the arms and shoulders.

and they do not hang around waiting for orders. Ultimately, however, they work as part of a finely tuned team, and their particular specialist skills will dovetail neatly with the skills of other members of that team.

Teamwork

Special Forces soldiers usually work in comparatively small groups and often operate far away from major army units. This situation means that the team members have to get to know each other extremely well and must cope with each other's foibles.

In certain observation activities, the members of a team may all occupy a small space together for long periods of time. There is little variation in the routine, there is nothing much to distinguish night from day, the food is boringly predictable and nothing much happens for a long time. In these circumstances, it would be disastrous if there were a clash of personalities or if someone could not control himself.

Self-Discipline

Many of the specialist trades carried out by Special Forces require a high degree of self-control. If you are involved in target acquisition, you may have to wait for days for anything to happen. If you are a sniper, you will have to calculate each movement with infinite care and

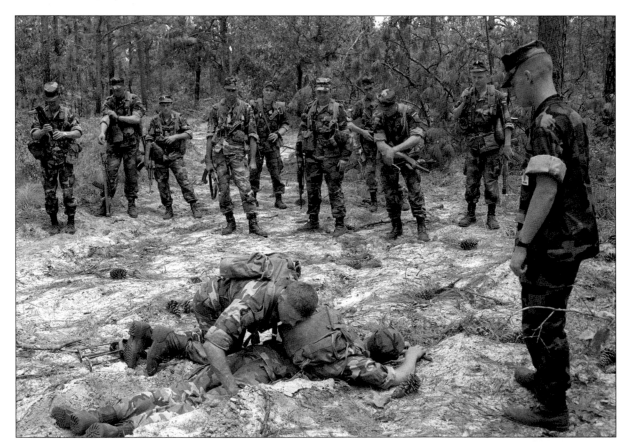

Above: Recruits learn how to check a 'body' for hidden items or weapons. Well-tried techniques become second nature and maximize efficiency and safety.

can spend hours moving across just a few feet of ground. Infinite patience is also required in travelling through the jungle brush to avoid being seen or heard by the enemy.

The Special Forces soldier owes it to himself as well as his team to be absolutely reliable with his equipment. Special Forces soldiers do not leave buttons undone so that kit can fall out, or forget to clean their weapons so that they jam at the vital moment. They do not wait to be beasted by a sergeant major in order to maintain the highest standards of personal and equipment readiness. They cannot afford to have a quiet snooze when nobody is looking when they are on observation duty.

Motivation

To get through training courses that even highly trained and experienced regular soldiers cannot manage requires an extremely high degree of motivation. Inevitably, somewhere along the line the thought 'What's the point?' will keep coming into your mind.

The motivation that keeps you going with a pack rubbing on your shoulders and your legs aching is the same motivation that may save your life in a survival situation.

Pressure

A Special Forces soldier needs to think on his feet when he is very tired and under pressure. Special training should prepare you for the kind of pressure that could exist in a war, where bombs are dropping, bullets are flying and nothing appears to be happening according to the book. The ability to stay calm in such circumstances and to continue to be effective is what marks out the Special Forces soldier from the run-of-the-mill trooper. Individuals who can remain calm in such circumstances can impose their plans on even the most chaotic

circumstances. When the chips are down and the enemy appears to hold all the cards, the Special Forces soldier will have the aggressive determination required to turn the tables.

Tenacity

Tenacity is the limpet-like determination not to give up even when all the observable evidence dictates that you should. It is a quality beyond positive thinking. Tenacity is a hard-boiled core that keeps glowing and functioning when your other physical and mental systems have all but closed down. To develop tenacity, you need to prove it to yourself, in your own training regimes and through the dark and difficult moments of doubt when there seems to be no light at the end of that tunnel.

Selflessness

It is one thing getting yourself through a training course, but quite another helping someone else through. Extreme training will literally bind a team together. Log races will demonstrate that when you fail, the team fails. Instructors on Special Operations courses are looking for people who not only have the ability to get themselves through, but also to help other people and, if necessary, literally carry them.

Reliability and Composure

You may well be a tough guy while out on the hills, but can you be that same tough guy while cramped up in a small space for days at a time or having to undergo capture and interrogation? Even in simulation, being taken captive and having your freedom denied places severe psychological pressure on the individual. You may sit for hours in a cold room with a sack over your head. You may also be interrogated.

In these circumstances a Special Forces soldier has to maintain his presence of mind,

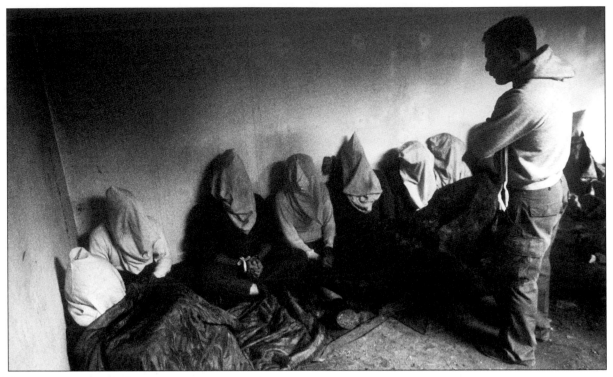

Above: In this simulated training exercise, a member of a 'terrorist' force interrogates hooded captives. Hooding can be extremely disorienting, which is why training for this possible scenario is so important for Special Forces troops.

even when being humiliated and having the same questions asked of him over and over again.

In these circumstances the successful candidate is likely to be the one who is capable of turning his system on to 'slow burn', keeping a core of who he is and what he is about deep down inside himself, while his exterior appears grey and of little consequence.

Intelligence and Common Sense

It goes without saying that a Special Forces soldier needs intelligence to deal with a bewildering array of problems, often while operating sophisticated machinery. He requires a high degree of battlefield awareness and may be responsible for bringing down artillery or aircraft fire through the use of sophisticated codes, while ensuring he does not wipe out either his own unit or friendly forces. A Special Forces soldier needs to be able to size up fast-changing scenarios very quickly and to be able to think on his feet.

When something is not running according to plan, the elite soldier will have the common sense to discern what actions are appropriate in a given set of circumstances.

Humility

Humility is the virtue of self-knowledge. A Special Forces soldier knows what he is capable of, and he does not need to brag about it. He also knows his limitations. His capabilities are linked to an evenly balanced self-confidence. An elite soldier knows that he is at the peak of a training pyramid, but also that the sky and the stars are a long way above his head.

Vision

It has been said that every soldier carries a field marshal's baton in his knapsack. Vision is beyond focus, taking in the wider picture and the three-dimensional background. Vision may involve thinking where you want to be in five years' time; it may be an image of yourself having passed through arduous training. Vision is knowing that beyond the hard, muddy trail, the cold wind and the rain the sun is bound to come out at some point. Another thing about vision is that it has to be married to belief. You need to believe that you have a part to play in the scenario that you envisage. You need not only to see yourself in that green, red or fawn beret, but also to believe that it is really you that the cap fits and that you will go on from strength to strength. If you do not believe, then your vision will remain two-dimensional or a scene in which you are impersonated by another character. You will need to test and strengthen your belief in order to make it real.

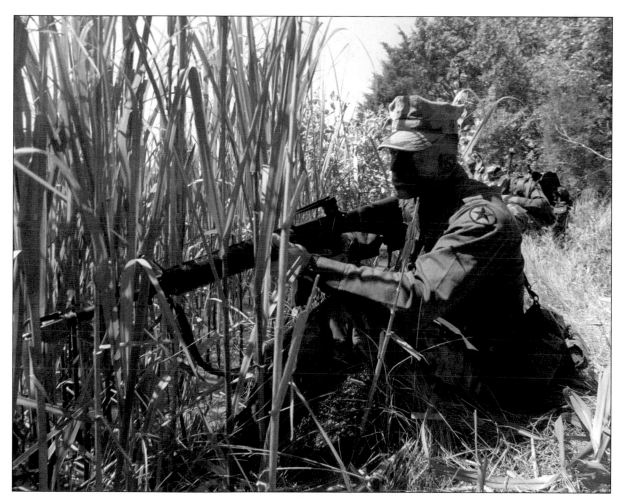

Above: Here, US Marine recruits undergo training in a riverine environment at Camp Le Jeune, North Carolina. Self-reliance and teamwork go hand-in-hand in all elite forces training. Each member of a group needs to be confident that the other is doing his job.

Thinking Skills

The power of our thoughts cannot be underestimated. You need to take your daily thoughts out of your mental wardrobe, dust them off and take a long, hard look at them. Then you need to decide which ones to keep and which ones to discard. There may be some thoughts that you have been hanging on to because you are rather attached to them, but they may not in fact be letting you down. A train of unhelpful thoughts frequently repeated will gradually seep into your subconscious and influence your attitude and view of reality. You will need to get yourself into the habit of thinking new and positive thoughts. It is said that it takes at least 30 days for anything to become habitual. Do not just promise yourself that you will change

your attitude. You need to keep repeating positive affirmations over and over again, until your conscious and subconscious mind accepts them as the new reality.

The more you acknowledge your own dignity as a human being and your abilities, the more your mind will seek to ensure that your circumstances fit with that positive self-image. There has to be a happy medium between being big-headed and beating yourself up over not being good enough. Once you have trained yourself to accept success with confidence, opportunities should begin to come your way.

Mental Imagery

Mental preparation for success should be part of your package of thinking skills. If you take the

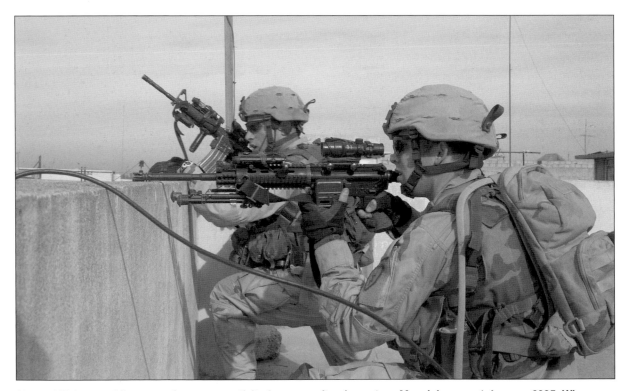

Above: US Army soldiers scan for enemy activity from a rooftop in eastern Mosul, Iraq, on 1 January 2005. When soldiers work together they provide mutual support and protection – here, when one soldier moves, the other is ready to provide covering fire.

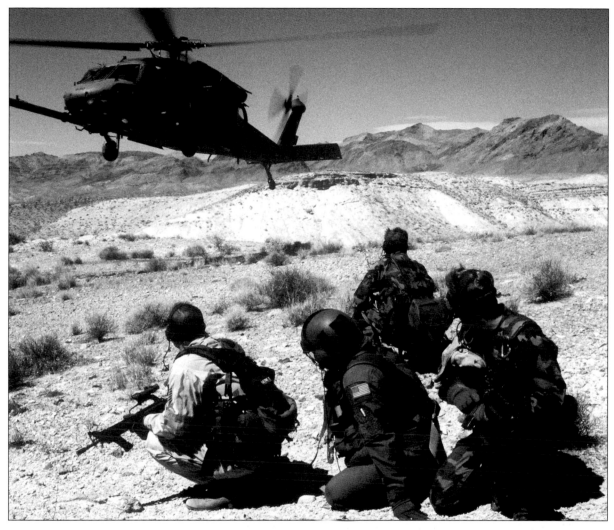

Above: US Special Forces are picked up by a Sikorsky MH-60K Black Hawk helicopter in the Somalian desert, 1992. In such circumstances, soldiers have to rely on their own resourcefulness to survive.

time to prepare yourself for likely eventualities, they will be less likely to catch you out. Instead, therefore, of being distracted by the unexpected, you will be more likely to remain calm and focused on your goals. No one can see into the future, and you have to make allowances for unexpected setbacks.

Yet if your calm attitude is predetermined, distractions are far less likely to put you off. If you take time to learn from past mistakes and rehearse in your mind how you are going to get it right next time, your whole performance should flow much more successfully in reality.

Mental imagery is similar to carrying out a physical practice without being physically present. It is true that you cannot replace actual practice in any activity, but running through the sequence of events mentally will mean that your mind is engaged and prepared when the event happens in reality.

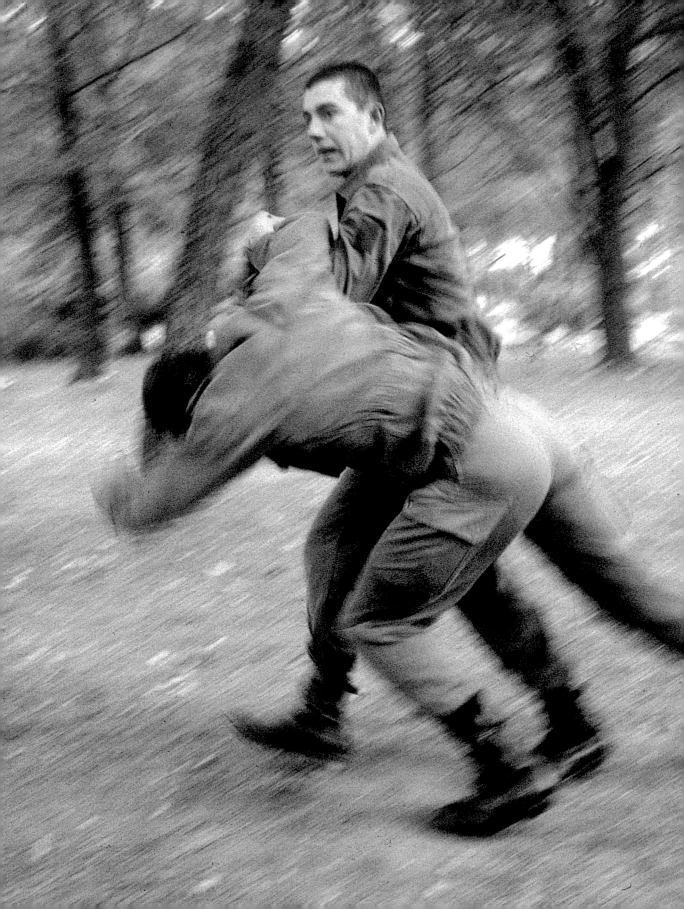

CHAPTER FIVE

Defeating an Opponent

Real elite forces soldiers are far removed from the image of Rambo. In order to do their job effectively, they spend much of their time keeping out of enemy contact. When they engage, it is with incisive expertise and after careful planning.

Elite forces are trained to have a high grade of awareness of their surroundings. The likelihood is that if you are in the presence of a Special Forces soldier in a crowded place, although he may not be looking at you, he is aware of your presence, has sized up your potential as a threat and will be ready to take action if you should approach him aggressively.

Even though highly trained, an elite forces soldier does not want to get involved in any form of personal combat unless it cannot be avoided. However skilful he may be at defending himself, a scuffle with a drunk, bully or mugger is always going to attract attention, as well as the possibility of injury.

Do Not Invite Attack

Potential assailants want to find a victim who is least likely to resist. Just as animals have a sixth sense that tells them which animal in a herd is the weakest, humans also instinctively pick up certain clues from a person's behaviour that attract their attention.

A bully needs to show off in front of an audience in order to raise his fragile self-image, and he will not run the risk of picking on a strong

Opposite: French Foreign Legion soldiers practise unarmed combat techniques in a forest setting. Such methods require professional training and are governed by strict military law.

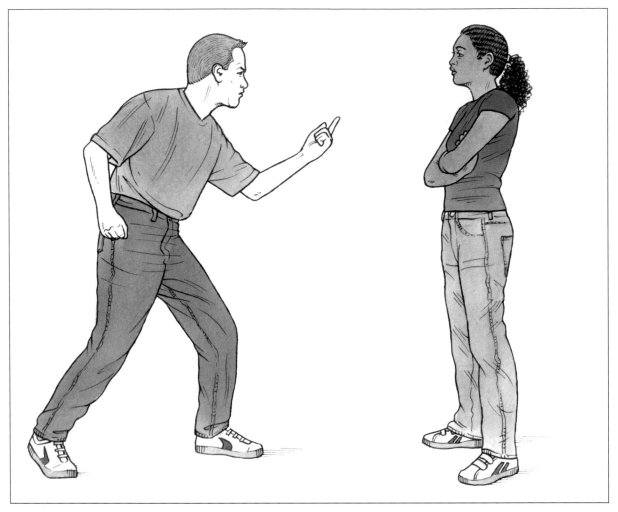

Above: In the face of a potential attack, a confident, upright stance is more likely to deter threatening behaviour. Maintaining a calm, controlled exterior will best help you to deal with the situation.

person who might retaliate and make him look foolish. A bully will look out for the following signs of weakness:

1. Rounded or hunched shoulders, or a manner of walking that suggests the person's head is sinking into the shoulders like a tortoise's into its shell.
2. A weak, tentative smile that shows an eagerness to please, rather than a confident view of the world.
3. Eyes looking down at the ground. Shifting eyes which dart about and seem unable to rest on any particular spot.
4. Crossed arms and legs, suggesting evasive self-protection by minimizing the area of visible body surface.
5. Detachment from a peer group and a lack of any verbal or physical signs of bonding with that group.
6. Difficulty in responding to challenging remarks.

7. High or uncertain pitch or timbre in the voice; hesitant way of talking.
8. Hands hovering around the face area.

You can do a great deal to reduce the likelihood of being targeted as a potential victim, either when you are walking down the street or among gatherings of people:

1. Improve your physical strength and overall conditioning through exercise. This produces numerous benefits. You will be physically

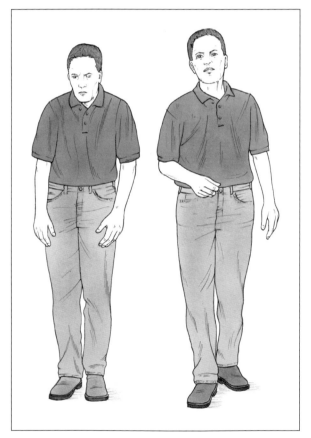

Above: Examples of poor posture (left) and good posture (right). Sagging shoulders and eyes looking at the ground suggest lack of self-respect. Keeping your shoulders back and walking confidently is more likely to deter potential assailants.

stronger and your posture will improve from a fuller chest, squarer shoulders, upright back and that natural poise and balance that comes from well-conditioned muscles. Your physical condition will mean that you have both the strength to stand and fight if absolutely necessary and the ability to outrun your assailant and get out of danger. Notice that lions in the Serengeti pick on the animals which are least likely to be able to outrun them. Your physical fitness will also have side effects on the timbre of your voice – developed lungs and a strong abdomen produce stronger sounds. Your physical strength will also give you more confidence in difficult situations.

2. Make sure your gaze is steady and straight ahead. You will be surprised by how much

POSTURE

The easiest way to achieve good posture is by taking regular exercise. If your body is conditioned through exercise – which may involve running plus some upper-body exercise such as moderate weight training – your muscles will hold your frame in its optimum stance, with a straight back, shoulders back and neck straight. Well-balanced muscles and correct posture will produce a natural grace of movement and improve your balance and agility.

The side effect of regular exercise is that your confidence in yourself is also likely to be improved and you are likely to transmit an aura of assurance. You are, in fact, a force to be reckoned with and therefore less likely to be victimized.

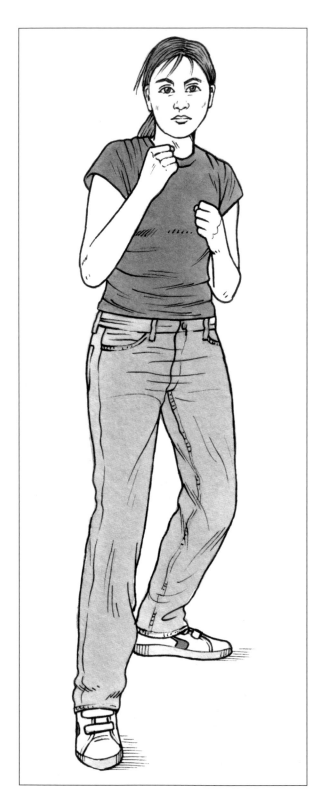

Left: If you are physically threatened, the on-guard position provides you with optimum balance on your feet, with one leg forward and the other leg behind, knees slightly bent. The hands are raised to deflect a blow to the face or upper body and to respond if necessary. The leading hand is higher than the other. Forward movement is begun with the leading leg. The stance is maintained throughout the period of threat.

you can see without darting your eyes to left and right, or turning your head. A potential assailant may be staring at you to catch your eye, and you are much more likely to catch his if your eyes are darting around uncertainly. Practise your peripheral vision with a friend – see how much visual information you can pick up as they move to the edge of your vision. If an activity is suspicious and you want to follow it, move your head slightly as if to focus on a new point still ahead of you. By pretending not to notice you will retain an element of surprise, as you will move when your assailant does not expect it.

3. Keep a measured expression on your face. If you are going to smile, do so in a definite manner for good reason. Otherwise keep your mouth level in a neutral, open expression.

4. If sitting, keep both feet flat on the floor, and with your upper legs placed evenly, the knees neither together nor too wide apart. Keep your hands in your lap or on any bag you may have, or on top of a table. If you are standing, keep your legs evenly apart on the ground and your hands by your side.

5. If you are with a group, contribute and join in, and also remain with them if necessary.

6. Speak steadily, remembering to take air fully into your abdomen. Fear and anxiety tend to constrict breathing, so you may need to make a conscious physical effort to fill your solar plexus. Speak calmly and slowly, placing

emphasis where necessary. If you are exchanging remarks, do not be roused by brash or insulting statements, but continue to say what you want to say.

7. If you are walking, walk purposefully and steadily, but not hurriedly. Keep your shoulders back. Sometimes slowing your pace can have a very disconcerting effect on any potential pursuer. The last thing a pursuer expects is for the person they are following to slow down. The effect is similar with animals: firm, confident movements reassure animals or deter barking dogs that may have a mind to taking a snap at you. Hurried, worried movements tend to confirm your victim status.

8. Always be aware of your surroundings, as well as the people around you. Anyone who glances at you and moves out of your peripheral vision may be about to come up behind you. Get your timing right and make your escape if the need arises. Keep an eye out for possible allies.

Self-Defence

If you are physically attacked by an aggressor you have the right to use proportionate force to defend yourself. You may need to prove that the force you used was not disproportionate, especially if the aggressor sustained an injury.

To find out about self-defence, you should consult the relevant reputable books or qualified

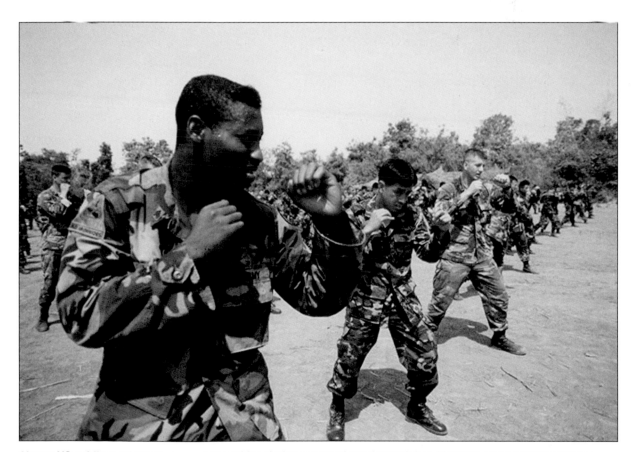

Above: US soldiers adopt the on-guard position during unarmed combat training. Methods employed by military personnel, however, cannot be used by civilians.

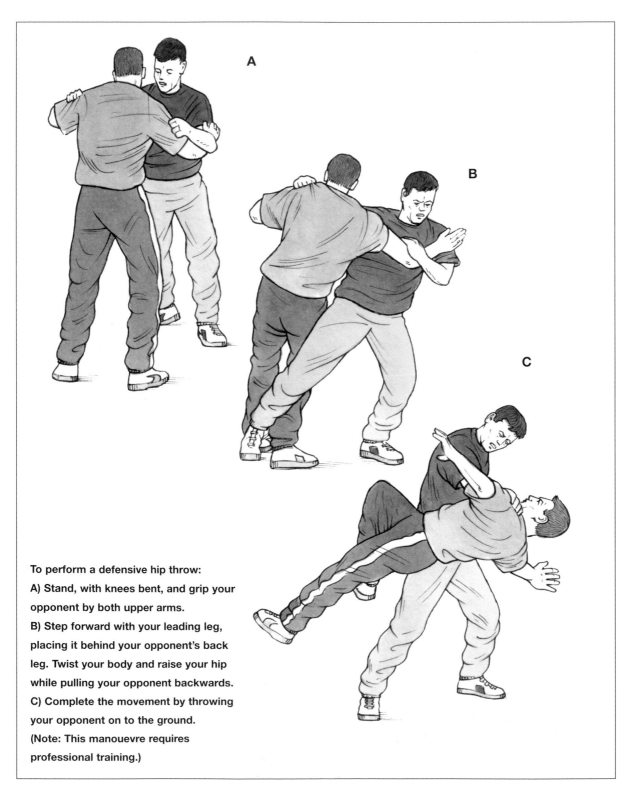

A

B

C

To perform a defensive hip throw:

A) Stand, with knees bent, and grip your opponent by both upper arms.

B) Step forward with your leading leg, placing it behind your opponent's back leg. Twist your body and raise your hip while pulling your opponent backwards.

C) Complete the movement by throwing your opponent on to the ground.

(Note: This manouevre requires professional training.)

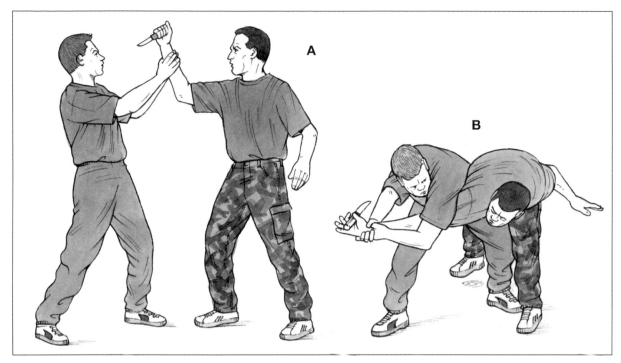

Above: If someone attempts to stab you with a knife, grab their forearm with both hands and, holding their wrist firmly with both hands (A), twist your body round and force their arm down across your right knee, placing your left leg between their legs (B).

trainers. If you are a civilian, you should put up the most effective defence that will allow you to escape unharmed. It should be stated that, although you may have studied self-defence tactics in books or even learned them in training sessions, a real-life assault may not allow you time to practise skilful moves; you may be paralysed with fear or your attacker may do something entirely unpredictable – in short, the attacker will not have read the script.

It is important, therefore, to practise a few simple but reliable moves thoroughly until they are almost second nature.

Competitive Behaviour

Your aim if you wish to become an elite soldier is not to beat someone else, but to do and be your best. If you get tied up with trying to do better than a particular individual, or get into negative behaviour trying to keep them in their place, it will distract you from your primary goal.

Competition, when used correctly, can help you. If there is someone who is on a similar level to you mentally and physically, that person can help you to raise your standard to compete with him. If you are on the receiving end of negative, competitive behaviour, the best tactic is to remain focused on your goal. Such behaviour often arises when the other person feels threatened by your natural gifts and talents. They may, therefore, do their best to undermine you. Do not respond emotionally to their tactics, but remain calm and focused on your goal.

If you allow yourself to be drawn into a wrangle with the other person, or if you show anger, it will only mean that they have found

COMPETING – WITH YOURSELF

Rather than competing with other people and thereby giving yourself a temporary sense of false security if you win, or damaging your confidence if you lose, it is better to focus on doing your best with the mental and physical equipment you have. Knowing you have done your best will provide you with greater long-term satisfaction and confidence. You can achieve your potential by setting realistic goals and committing to them.

ways to push your buttons and control your behaviour. There is nothing more exasperating than being ignored, especially in this case, and your antagonist should start to back off when he sees that he is making no impression and that you are continuing to achieve.

If your competitor undermines you in some way that might affect your position, you can as a first step warn them personally (do not get into a 'discussion' if there is nothing to discuss; they may want to get into something that is none of their business). If they do not heed the warning, take the problem up with a person in authority. If he or she cannot see your point of view, take it higher. If you find no resolution, stay strong and either keep going in your current job or look for another one.

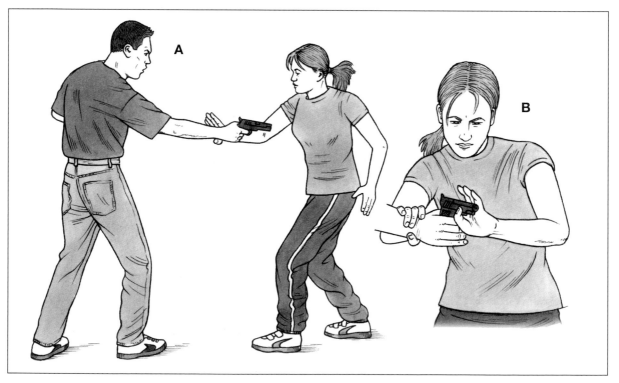

Above: To defend against an assailant with a handgun, strike out and push the inside of the assailant's gun arm away from your body (A), then use the other hand to grasp the gun and twist the weapon away from yourself and out of his or her hand. (Note: This manoeuvre should be performed only by a professionally trained person.)

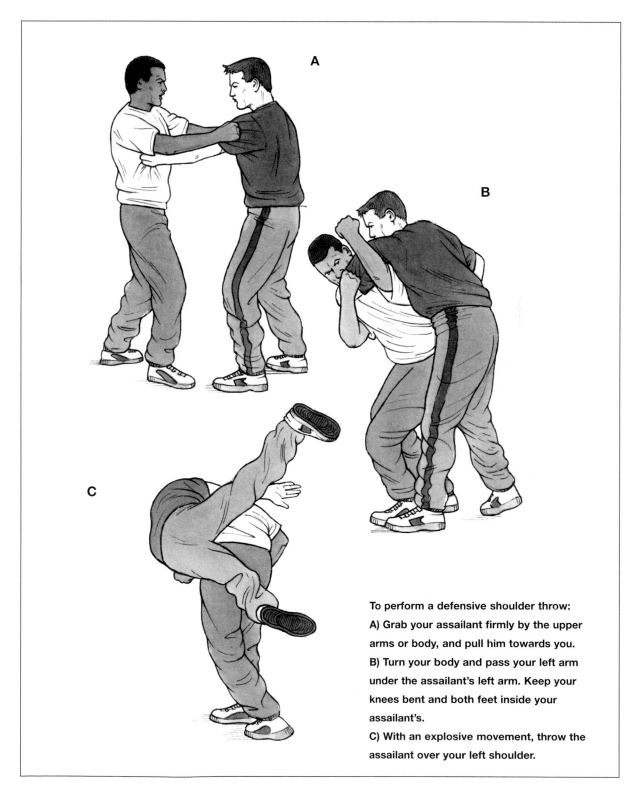

A

B

C

To perform a defensive shoulder throw:
A) Grab your assailant firmly by the upper arms or body, and pull him towards you.
B) Turn your body and pass your left arm under the assailant's left arm. Keep your knees bent and both feet inside your assailant's.
C) With an explosive movement, throw the assailant over your left shoulder.

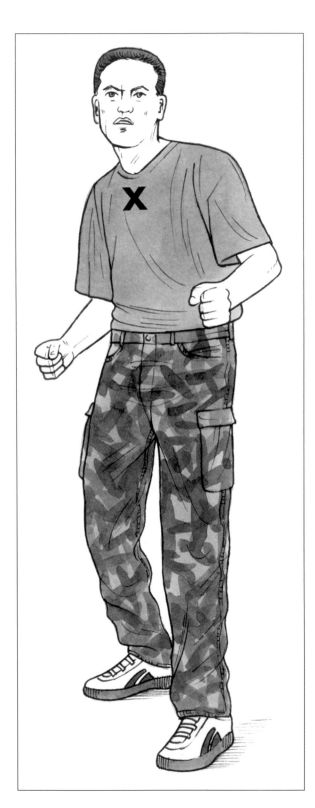

Left: When under physical threat, you should maintain your focus on a point just below your assailant's collarbone. This will maximize your awareness of any movement in his arms without allowing you to be distracted by what he might be saying.

Taking Advantage

You will have the advantage if you have a plan and are focused on your interim goals, as well as holding a vision for the future. You will have the advantage if you focus on the 'controllables' – in other words, the things that you can change. Those things relate to your thoughts, your choices, your behaviour and your standards.

Other people cannot control those things unless you allow them to do so. You will have the advantage if you recognize that not everything is controllable. Once you have acknowledged the likelihood of difficulties and surprises, you will be better prepared to deal with them. Most of all, you will have the advantage if you are the one with the powers of endurance.

Ultimately, although we function largely in teams, partnerships and communities, we have full responsibility for our individual attitudes and behaviour. Teams function efficiently when individuals carry out their own tasks professionally, and this may require a certain degree of autonomy, initiative and a proactive attitude. By developing a healthy sense of autonomy, you can feel confident in your own achievements and you are better placed to appreciate the achievements of others.

Opposite: To perform a defensive side kick:
A) Turn to one side and raise and coil one leg.
B and C) Uncoil the raised leg explosively into your assailant's midriff. Strike the assailant with the side of your foot and twist the hips.
(Note: These moves can be classified as assault unless they are used in proven cases of self-defence.)

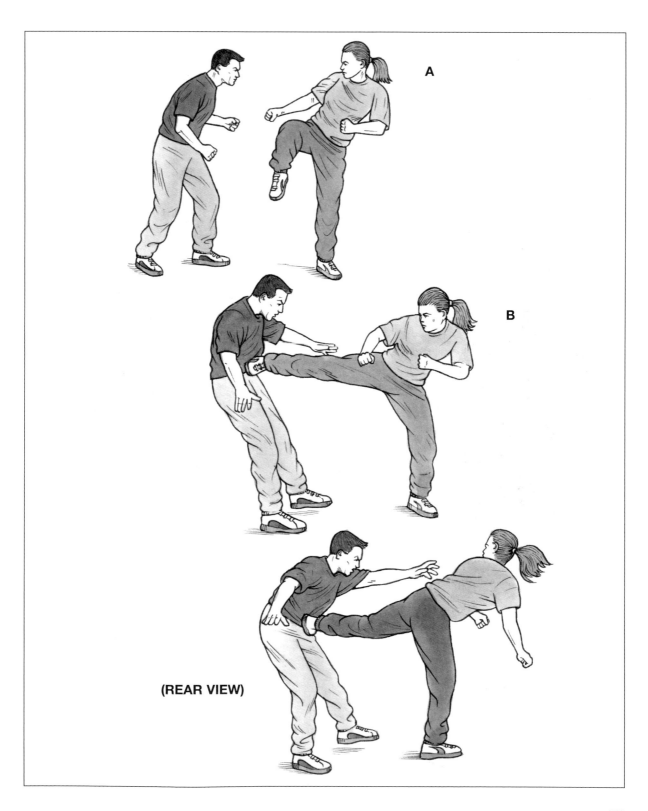

A

B

(REAR VIEW)

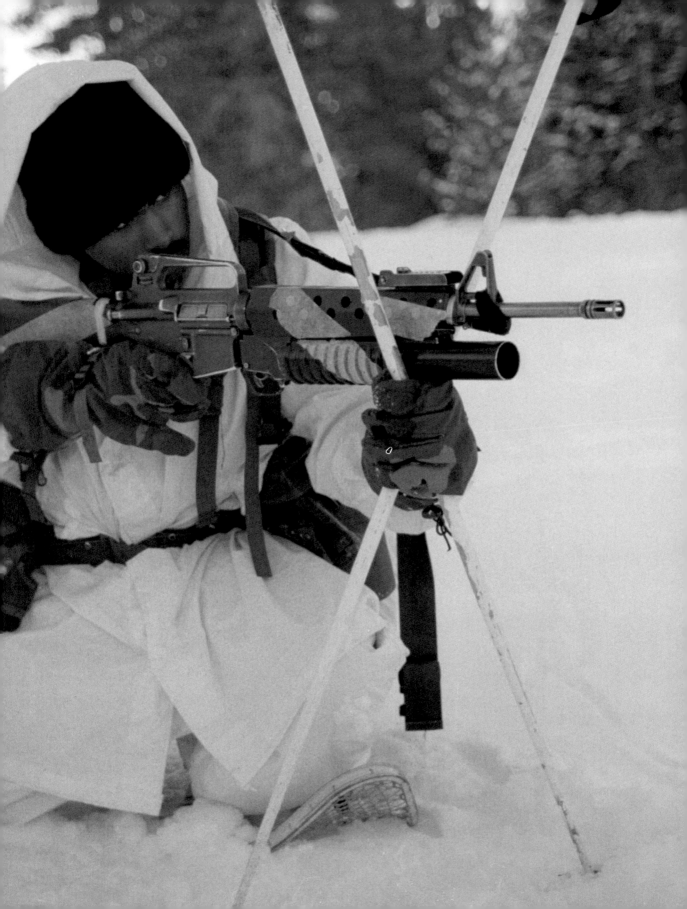

CHAPTER SIX

Advanced Techniques

Part of the training of the elite forces soldier is adaptation to and survival in different environments. If a soldier is fighting the elements or suffering from either hypothermia or dehydration, he will not be able to carry out his tasks efficiently.

It is often said that you should know your enemy. Although nature certainly contains beautiful places, it is also extremely tough. If it is not treated with the proper respect, nature will get the better of you. Special Forces soldiers have training regimes that take them through desert regions, the tropics, waterways and seas, and cold and mountainous regions.

Endurance in Deserts

US and British armed forces, along with various allies, have fought two recent major wars in the Middle East, and in the interim have been based for long periods in desert regions on varying stages of alert. Special Operations forces have famously been inserted into enemy territory in desert regions both in Iraq and in Afghanistan, calling on a high level of endurance in these challenging environments.

Desert regions are characterized by less than 25cm (10in) of annual rainfall, an evaporation rate that exceeds precipitation and a high average temperature. Perennial plants are restricted to water courses and other wet areas, and no cultivation is possible unless the land is reclaimed in some way. The high pressure over

Opposite: Advanced techniques enable soldiers to operate efficiently in extreme temperatures. Soldiers need to master the environment if they are to master their enemy.

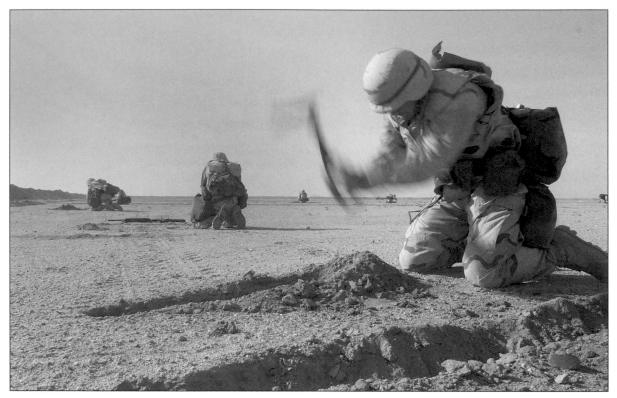

Above: Hard work in the heat of the desert, such as digging a shell-scrape, requires physical fitness and must be backed up by adequate supplies of food and, most especially, water.

deserts means that rain is sparse, irregular and unpredictable. Low humidity in the atmosphere allows sunlight to penetrate directly during the day, with temperatures reaching up to 55°C (131°F) in the shade. As sand does not retain heat, the heat is lost rapidly at nightfall and temperatures can quickly drop to near freezing. The temperature range may be 30°C (86°F), and there can even be frost and snow in the winter.

The lack of vegetation in deserts means the soil is easily affected by wind and the occasional appearance of water. Water can sometimes rush down from hilly areas to form canyons. Whether it is rock, sand, salt marsh or wadi, a desert is hard work to traverse. The Empty Quarter is so called because even the local Bedouin tribesmen know better than to try to cross it.

Clothing
Clothing should be lightweight, although it needs to provide enough protection from the direct effects of sunlight or the effects of sand. Sand reflects sunlight much like glass, and the effects can be countered either by sand goggles or by the use of an Arab headdress, which is wrapped around the head. A neckerchief or handkerchief can also be placed over the nose and mouth, and tied behind the head.

Footwear
Footwear should be light and breathable, and have a sole thick enough to resist the heat of the daytime sand. Care must be taken to keep sand out of the inside of the boot, as sand is highly abrasive and can cause blisters.

DESERT REGIONS

There are more than 50 major deserts spread across the world, from North America and the African continent to Asia and Australasia. Some of the world's major deserts include:

● ATACAMA (363,000 square kilometres; 140,000 square miles)
This is a litoral desert located in northern Chile. It runs down a narrow belt between the Andes Mountains and the Pacific Ocean. The region has little vegetation and the mean annual precipitation is around 10cm (4in).

● GOBI DESERT (1,300,000 square kilometres; 501,800 square miles)
The Gobi Desert in based on a plateau fringed by mountains. The height of the plateau ranges from 914m (3000ft) above sea level in the east to 1542m (5000ft) above sea level in the west. Made up mostly of gravel plains, the Gobi contains a mixture of grass, scrub and thorn over three-quarters of its extent, with occasional wells and shallow lakes. The southeast area is waterless.

● GREAT SANDY DESERT (360,000 square kilometres; 140,000 square miles)
Situated between the Pilbara and Kimberley rocky ranges, the Great Sandy Desert is made up of sand and rock, with some desert vegetation. Temperatures range between more than 32°C (90°F) in January to 10°–15°C (50°–60°F) in July.

● GREAT VICTORIA DESERT (647,000 square kilometres; 250,000 square miles)
Australia's Great Victoria consists largely of a terrain of sandhills, grasslands and salt lakes.

Temperatures range from 32°–40°C (90°–104°F) in summer to 18°–23°C (64°–75°F) in winter.

● KALAHARI DESERT (500,000 square kilometres; 193,000 square miles)
The Kalahari is an arid to semi-arid desert, with large swathes of reddish soil with grasses and brush and sand to the east. It also contains some major game reserves and is inhabited by the famous Bushmen people, who are a living testament to human survival in difficult conditions. The Kalahari is bounded by the Orange and Okavango rivers.

● MOJAVE DESERT (38,850 square kilometres; 15,000 square miles)
The Mojave is bordered to the north and west by the Sierra Nevada and the Tehachapi, San Gabriel and San Bernardino mountains. To the southeast it merges with the Colorado desert. It has typical desert vegetation and is interspersed with lakes and streams. The Mojave was once an inland sea and was formed by volcanic activity.

● RUB AL KHALI, OR EMPTY QUARTER (582,750 square kilometres; 225,000 square miles)
This desert comprises the largest area of continuous sand in the world and occupies more than a quarter of Saudi Arabia. Sand dunes in the Empty Quarter rise to a level of about 200m (660ft), and the desert as a whole is about 1005m (3300ft) above sea level in the west, sloping down to about sea level in the east. Although extremely dry and practically uninhabited, the Empty Quarter contains important oil reserves and some of the world's largest oil fields.

SAND MARATHON

Although a civilian event, the Marathon des Sables incorporates many of the lessons learned in this book and is at the high end of the kind of endurance achievements that elite forces personnel would be proud of.

The course is 140 miles (230 km) across the Moroccan desert in heat that can rise to 38°C (100°F). The terrain is a mix of sand, dunes, stony flats, hills, dried lakes and the occasional palm grove. A typical seven-day itinerary in the marathon breaks down as:

Day 1 – 28km (17.5 miles)
Day 2 – 35km (22 miles)
Day 3 – 38km (24 miles)
Day 4 – 77km (48 miles)
Day 5 – rest day
Day 6 – 42km (26 miles)
Day 7 – 18km (11 miles)

Contestants find themselves negotiating a succession of sand dunes 60m (200ft) high, and probably with a Saharan wind blowing a large

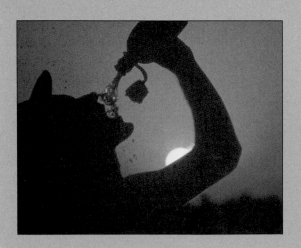

amount of sand in their faces. The contestants are also required to carry all necessary food and equipment while racing, and this has to be carefully measured so that no excess weight is carried without detriment to fluid and nutritional requirements. It recommended high-energy snacks are eaten at least every thirty minutes throughout the race, and the day is sandwiched between a substantial breakfast and supper.

The organizers recommend a calorific intake of 15 per cent animal and vegetable proteins in order to maintain nitrogen balance; 30 per cent of the daily intake should be fat; 55 per cent of the calorie intake should be carbohydrate, divided between rapid-burn sugar and slow-burn sugar found in pasta, bread, potatoes and rice. They also recommend 1 to 1.5ml of water per calorie ingested, amounting to between six and seven litres per day. On top of all this, the recommendation is to add electrolytes and vitamins, including potassium, calcium, phosphorous, magnesium, and vitamins C, B1, B2 and PP.

As recommended elsewhere in this book, dried fruits and nuts or energy bars are suggested as regular snacks throughout the race, and an energy drink with glucose is also recommended at the end of each day to aid revitalization of the body.

The clothing recommendations are almost identical to the those adopted by the native Berbers – in other words, loose-fitting cotton that allows air to pass round the body and which is unlikely to chafe. This recommendation may come as a surprise to those used to high-tech clothing solutions.

Water

Water is a priority in the desert for obvious reasons. If you have plenty of both food and water, do not neglect solid nutrition just because the heat makes you feel less hungry. If you are short of water, however, your food consumption should take second place to your water consumption, as solid food absorbs water in the stomach during the digestive process. Foods rich in fat require more water to break down than foods rich in carbohydrates or proteins. Fruit requires very little water to digest. If water is short, make sure you work out a sensible ration early on, then stick to it, because lack of water may affect your ability to make this kind of judgment at a later stage.

In a temperate climate, an adult will lose about 1.5 litres (3½ US pints / 2¾ UK pints) of water per day through sweating, breathing and urinating. In a hot climate, this figure rises to 2–5 litres (4½–11¼ US pints / 3½–9 UK pints). If hard physical exertion is involved the figure may be 10 litres (21½ US pints / 17½ UK pints). When walking in a temperature of more than 38°C (100°F), you will be losing about 1 litre (2¼ US pints / 1¾ UK pints) per hour.

To conserve water and minimize dehydration, it is better to stay under cover during the hottest part of the day and do any work in the evening, night and morning. If you are short of water, you can take advantage of the natural dew at night by building a simple solar still.

Building a Solar Still

You will need a 0.5m (6ft) square plastic sheet, a container, a drinking tube and a rock. First dig a hole approximately 1m (3ft) across and about 0.6m (2ft) deep in an unshaded spot.

Dig another hole for the container at the bottom of the hole. The wider the container, the more water it is likely to catch.

Place one end of a tube in the container and the pass the other end up to the lip of the hole.

Stretch the plastic sheet over the hole, covering the edges with soil to anchor it. The sheet should droop into the hole about 40cm (16in), the lowest point of the dip being above the container.

Put a fist-sized stone at the centre of the sheet, directly above the container. Make sure that the sheeting does not touch the side of the hole, otherwise the earth will absorb the condensed water. Within 24 hours there should be about 1 litre (2¼ US pints / 1¾ UK pints) of water. The process of distillation makes the water safe to drink. You should drink the water through the straw.

One still will not, however, provide enough water for survival. If this is to be your main source of water, try to make sure you have three or four stills going at the same time, if you have access to the necessary materials.

In the desert you can also search for water in the following places or using the following signs:
- dried-up gulleys and water courses (dig down at the lowest point or the outside of a bend).
- animal tracks or droppings may well lead you to water and you can also follow the line of flight of birds.
- look for any sign of greenery.
- clouds, rain or lightning will signal the fall of rain.
- the foot of cliffs or rocks – water sometimes collects in depressions or holes.
- caves and fissures – you can probe these with a tube.
- any signs of a well or man-made structures.

Plants Containing Water

Cactus: cut off the top of a barrel cactus and extract the pulp. Mash the pulp and suck the water out.

- Date palm: cut a lower branch near the base and liquid should start to ooze out of the cut.
- Baobab tree: water is collected in the bulbous trunk during the rainy season.
- Prickly pears: both their fruit and ear lobes contain water.
- Saxaul: the spongy bark contains water. Press the bark to extract the liquid.
- Roots: the bloodwood desert oak and water tree of Australia have roots near the surface. These can be cut and sucked to provide moisture.

Food

There is a variety of edible plants and animals in the desert, depending on which region of the world you are in. These include the abal, acacia, agave, baobab, date palm, desert amaranth, wild gourd, carob and prickly pear. Insects can be stripped down and cooked, and there is a variety of edible snakes and other reptiles.

If you are able to, carry an identification manual for poisonous snakes and other dangerous animals – do not attempt to approach poisonous varieties for food.

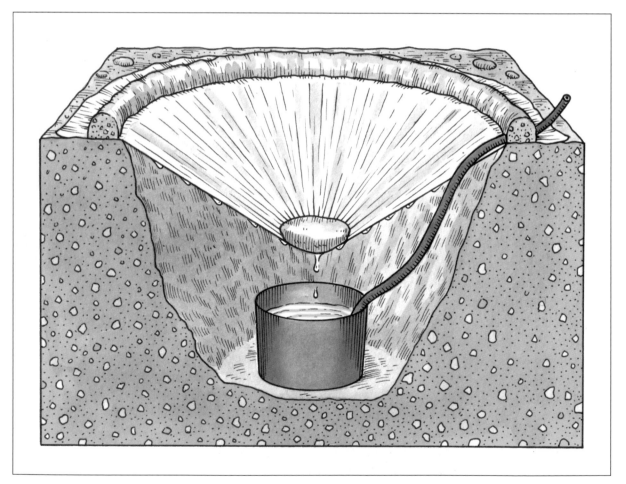

Above: To make a good solar still, a plastic sheet should be tightly sealed over a hole with a heavy stone placed in the centre. A tin placed in the centre of the hole will capture the condensation, while a tube or straw can be used to extract the water once it has gathered.

Endurance in Sea, River and Lake Systems

Many of the world's elite forces have a strong association with the sea and rivers, and their training will reflect this. Some units are part of their national naval command, for example, the United States Marine Corps and the British Royal Marines. Other units have Special Operations training in seaborne activities, such as the United States Navy SEALs and the British Special Boat Squadron (SBS).

Temperatures of surface water in the ocean range from 26°C (79°F) in tropical regions to -1.4°C (29.5°F), the freezing point for water, in polar regions. About 50 per cent of the world's oceans and seas have temperatures ranging between 1.3°C (29.5°F) and 3.8°C (39°F).

Water Safety

Any training in water involves danger. Whether you are plunging into the water from a helicopter or you are in a small assault boat, accidents can happen at any moment. In addition, in a live military engagement, your craft may be sunk by the enemy.

If your boat or ship is sunk and you are in the water, swim steadily and make for the nearest life raft. If there is no life raft, try to locate any piece of wreckage that might help with flotation. Should there be burning oil on the surface of the water, aim to swim upwind of the source of fire as soon as possible.

If you are surrounded by the burning oil, attempt to swim under it with strong strokes, trying to identify any clear patches where you

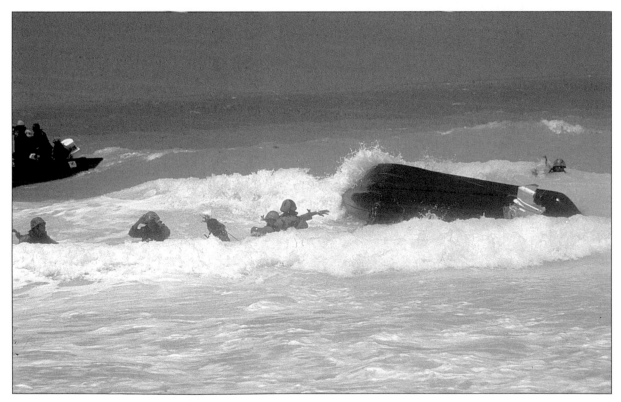

Below: A US Navy SEAL team struggles with heavy waves in a shoreside operation. By learning from mistakes in training, elite soldiers gradually hone their skills.

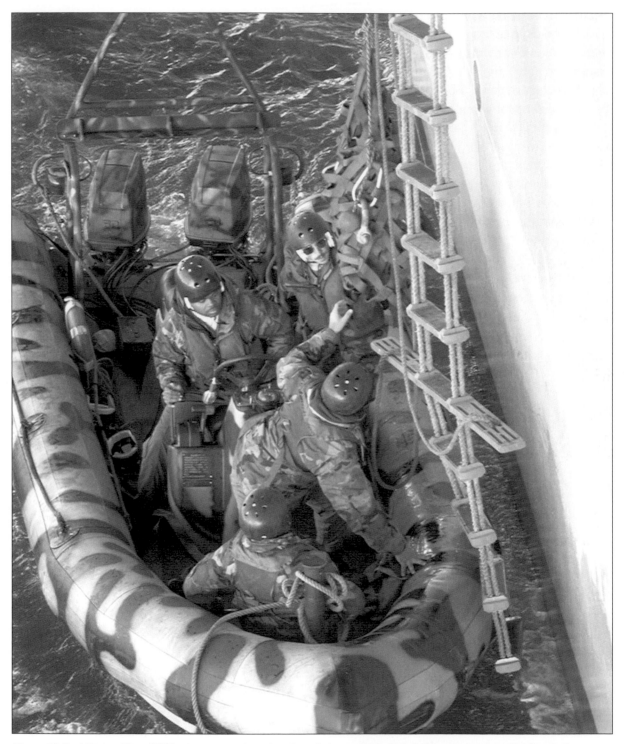

Above: United States Navy SEALs prepare to board a ship. Only continuous training can produce the level of efficiency required to carry out an assault unobserved, probably in the dark and perhaps in bad weather.

might come up for a breath (if you have a life jacket on, you may need to deflate it in order to get under the surface of the water). Once you come up in a clear patch, identify the next objective, take a good breath and submerge again, feet first.

Once you are away from immediate danger, your next priority is to conserve energy. You can

BOAT CRAFT

Elite forces such as the United States Navy SEALs or British Royal Marines are often required to carry out rapid insertions to and from beaches and other areas of the coastline. To do so effectively requires a thorough understanding of the powerful forces of nature involved, as well as the handling characteristics of the particular craft.

Natural conditions that must be considered include wind, tide and ocean currents, the depth of the sea, the gradient and composition of the beach, as well as obstacles such as rocks that could potentially capsize or sink a boat. Once a craft has been successfully beached, it must also be successfully withdrawn through the surf to be available for later recovery of personnel or other operations. In order to avoid being caught out, elite boat operators learn about the characteristics of surf, swell, breakers and wave troughs. They learn that the ideal landing area should be formed of sand and gravel.

As swells move towards a beach and encounter the upwardly sloping ocean floor, surf is created, first in the form of combers, then as breakers. Unfortunately for boat handlers, the surf does not follow a predictable pattern, even when the weather is calm, so the boat handler must always be ready for the unexpected.

As you approach the beach, do not be lulled into a false sense of security by the low level of the surf as you approach. Even tsunami waves can appear as no more than ripples when out at sea, and the same rule applies to surf. It will grow disproportionately as it approaches the shore. You should follow the surf line at right angles to its advance, bearing in mind that the surf line may not lie exactly parallel to the beach. Use a point on the beach as a marker.

● Try to pick up a sizeable wave as it passes under the boat and keep pace with it, just behind the crest.

● Hit the beach at speed and ensure the boat stays on the beach by using rudder and engines. The greatest danger at this point is 'broaching to', where the stern of the boat is thrown round by the force of the waves, and the boat is placed sideways-on to the surf and the beach. It could then be easily capsized or swamped.

● To return from the beach to the open sea, the craft should not be turned sideways on to the surf, unless it is small and light enough to be turned by hand while on the beach.

● When out at sea, head seas should be approached at a slight angle, between 15 and 45 degrees from head-on, as this can provide a smoother and safer ride.

● Likewise, take care of following seas, which can turn the boat stern-over-tip. It is better to try to ride on the back of a wave than to allow waves to keep pushing up behind the boat, which may also swamp it.

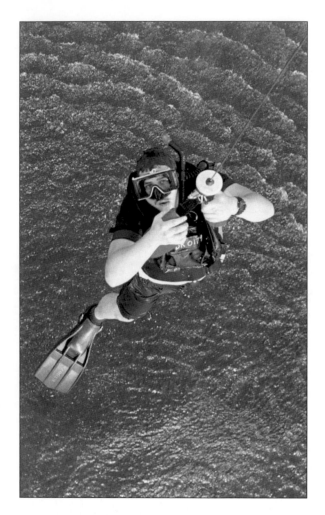

Left: A US Navy rescue swimmer is hoisted out of the sea by a CH-46D Sea Knight helicopter during a training exercise in the Red Sea. Rescue swimmers undergo comprehensive training in sea survival techniques.

If you have a life jacket, adopt the Heat Escaping Lessing Posture (HELP), which is designed to conserve as much warmth as possible. This means adopting a sitting position with legs crossed and the upper torso straight out of the water.

Life Raft

The recommended rescue procedures in a life raft include:

- Administer first aid, with priority for wounded survivors. Supply dry clothing where possible.
- Check for signalling equipment such as flares, emergency radio and flags. Take care to conserve batteries.
- Salvage any useful material.
- Ensure one member of the crew is attached to the life raft with a line, to prevent the raft blowing away in the event of a capsize.
- Institute water rationing.
- Check for desalting equipment and solar stills.
- Check available supplies of foods.
- Follow life-raft instructions, such as putting out a drogue.
- Paddle towards any other life rafts and attach a line of about 8m (25ft).
- If it is cold, huddle together for warmth.
- If it is hot and sunny, make sure some clothing is kept on, including hats, to protect against sunburn and sunstroke.

Rescue

If your boat has sunk, or aircraft ditched, rescue services will head for that area, so your task is to remain in the vicinity (if you are in a war scenario

try relaxing by floating on your back with your head above the surface of the water. Another way of conserving energy without a life jacket is to adopt a crouching position, whereby you take a breath of air, then relax with your head below the surface of the water, before bringing yourself up for more air. This saves you from the constant movement that is required to keep your head above water.

Some types of clothing can be used to enhance buoyancy, for example, by tying the end of a coat sleeve and blowing air into it. The process may need to be repeated, depending on the breathability of the fabric.

and in enemy territory, your priority is the opposite, so these rules do not apply). Military personnel will carry their own means of communication for rescue and follow their own instructions according to training.

General peacetime rescue procedures are as follows:

- Put out a sea anchor to remain close to the site. If you do not put out the anchor, the life raft will be carried away by the winds and the currents.
- Allocate tasks to everyone aboard, for example, signalling, fishing, navigating.
- Work out water rationing etc. at an early stage while your judgment is sound.
- Follow instructions for signalling equipment.
- Keep a log, recording wind, currents and the state of crew and supplies.

DANGEROUS MARINE LIFE

Operating in the world's oceans and seas may bring elite forces personnel into contact with some dangerous forms of marine life.

SHARKS

Shark attacks on humans range between 45 and 100 per year. The most dangerous species of shark are the great white shark, tiger shark, bull shark, oceanic white tip and the mako. Due to the power of large sharks, these attacks are often life-threatening or can result in the loss of limbs. A shark preparing to attack often swims with its pectoral fins pointing down and it begins to swim round its prey in ever-decreasing circles. Sharks are often attracted by blood, and they may also be alerted by panicky movements. As the shark is complete master of its environment, the best advice is to keep well away from them.

KILLER WHALES

There are no recorded attacks by killer whales on humans, but due to the potential lethality of an attack by such a large carnivorous marine animal, the advice, as with sharks, is to stay out of the water if they are present.

BARRACUDA

A barracuda, which can grow to 3m (10ft), is capable of delivering a nasty bite. Attacks are normally on surface swimmers and are unlikely to be life-threatening.

POISONOUS FISH

Divers may inadvertently touch or step upon a variety of poisonous fish that can deliver dangerous and painful – sometimes even lethal – stings. These include the weeverfish, stonefish, zebra-fish and scorpionfish, which have poisonous spines that are deployed when they are touched or disturbed. A stingray has a poisonous barb near the base of its tail, which can cause a painful wound.

CROCODILES, ALLIGATORS AND CAIMANS

All of these reptiles are extremely dangerous. Some of the most aggressive are thought to be saltwater crocodiles which inhabit estuaries. These are generally larger than the freshwater varieties. Extreme caution should be used wherever these animals might be present. They are also dangerous when on land, as they can run or lunge extremely swiftly.

Finding Land

If you are sure that there is no expectation of rescue near the accident site, you can try to make headway towards land. A life raft will be pushed by a mixture of water currents and wind. If it is light and high in the water, the effects of wind will be maximized. If it is heavy and low in the water, the effects of the water currents will be greater.

When you are relying most on wind power, it is a good idea to bring in the drogue and get rid of any unnecessary weight.

Indications of nearby land may include:

- A stationary cumulus cloud.
- Birds heading towards land in the afternoon and evening; they tend to head away from land in the morning.
- A light green reflection on the clouds above, which could be created by a lagoon.
- Floating vegetation or pieces of timber.

Once land is spotted, and if there is habitation on the land, make a signal and wait for rescue. If there is no sign of habitation, prepare to approach the land, taking care to avoid rocks or

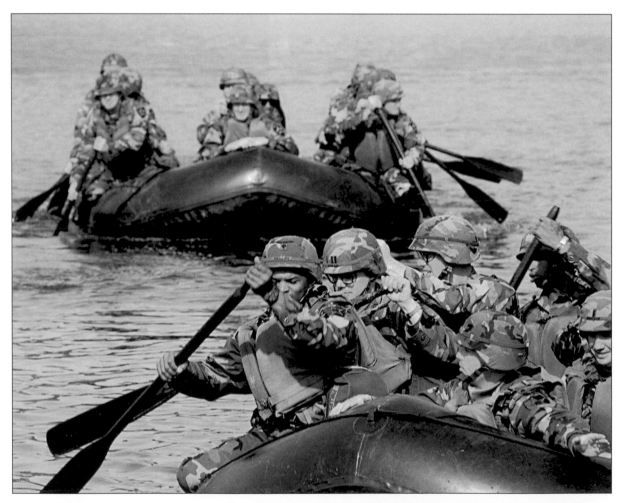

Above: A US Army engineer company paddle rubber rafts in Korea, 2000. Teamwork is maximised by continually working together. If each individual is doing their best, the team as a whole benefits.

RIVER OPERATIONS

Elite forces may deploy along jungle waterway in small boats, either powered by motors or using paddles, depending on the tactical scenario. Boats can be dropped into a river from a helicopter, with the personnel jumping afterwards. All the necessary equipment is lashed into the boat when it is dropped and the personnel just hold their personal weapons above their heads as they jump.

Jungle rivers may change after heavy rainfall and their banks are often covered with thick undergrowth which can easily conceal an enemy. Movement up river must, therefore, be carried out with extreme caution. When landing at a steep river bank, personnel exit the boat individually from the prow. If the landing place is flatter, personnel exit in twos. The two that are out of the boat provide covering fire for those that follow.

If not equipped with boats, soldiers may have to perform a river crossing with all their equipment. In these cases, the normal drill is to pack all dry clothing and boots into the rucksack or bergen, using a series of individual plastic bags to waterproof different items. The soldier will dress in his waterproof equipment to provide minimum protection during the crossing and perhaps use the rubber NBC (nucleur, biological and chemical) boots to provide necessary foot protection.

Depending on the rate of the current, the river crossing should be carried out from a point above the intended point of exit. If available, a rope can be slung across to the other bank and tied securely round a tree to provide guidance and safety.

Soldiers will follow individual unit recommendations on the stowage of weapons, though typically these will be attached to the packs and held out of the water. Some units make arrangements so that the weapons are readily accessible while in the water; others lash them more securely to the packs.

Soldiers cross in pairs, with the packs providing natural flotation throughout the crossing.

strong surf. Try to spot gaps in the surf (if you are approaching an island, try to get round to the lee shore, where it will be calmer), and attempt to locate a sloping beach, where the tide will be least strong. Should you be caught in a riptide, do not attempt to fight it, but wait for its energy to dissipate before attempting your approach once again.

Beware of coral reefs in the Pacific, as they are extremely sharp. When approaching a coral reef in a life raft, keep the drogue out for direction until you can judge the right distance and a suitably large wave to take you over the reef. Then take in the drogue in time to catch the wave.

Hang on to the craft at all times and wear as much protection as possible. If you are not in a raft, adopt a sitting position and keep your feet up as protection against any rocks.

Navigation without Instruments
Sunrise Method
The sun rises in the east and sets in the west. If you are north of latitude 23.5 degrees north, the

sun will pass to the south of you. If you are south of latitude 23.5 degrees south, the sun will pass to the north of you. Anywhere between these two latitudes, the sun's path will vary according to the time of year.

Watch Method

You can gain a rough estimate of your direction by using your watch between sunrise and sunset. Aim the hour hand at the sun and the point halfway between the hour hand and twelve o'clock will show the approximate direction of true south if you are in the northern hemisphere, and the approximate direction of true north if you are in the southern hemisphere. Note that this method is unreliable if you are in the tropical latitudes, between 23.5 degrees north and 23.5 degrees south.

The Stars

The North Star stands directly over the North Pole. This fact has saved many sailors' lives over the centuries. To identify the North Star, or Polaris, follow a line through the brightest stars

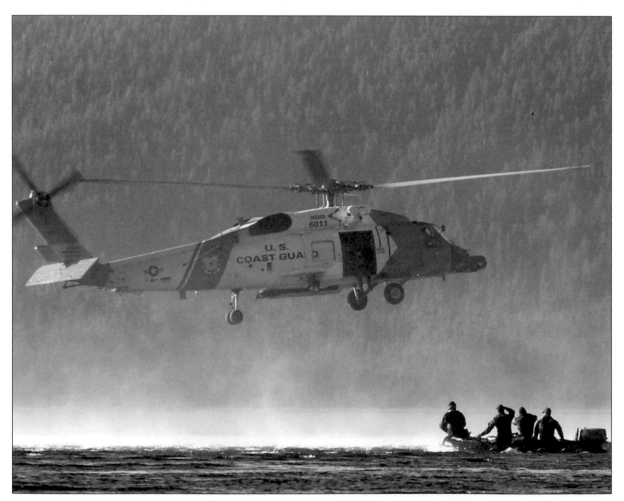

Above: A US Coast Guard helicopter hovers to pick up Navy SEALs in training. The successful recovery of service personnel is an important part of morale building.

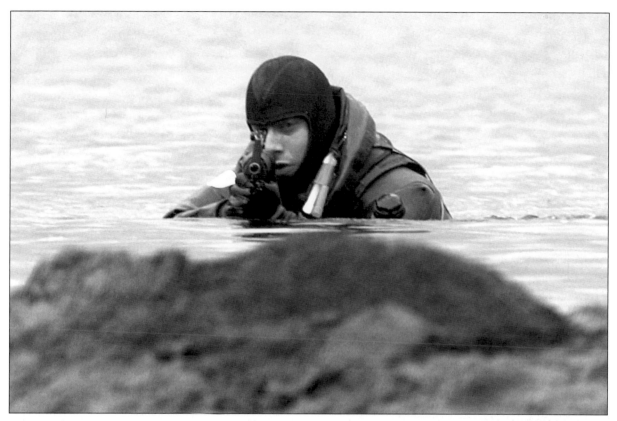

Above: A US special forces operative scans the shoreline as he conducts a beach reconnaissance in Sitka Bay, Alaska. Training exercises such as this allow soldiers to be mentally prepared for the challenges that they will be faced with in the field.

in the Ursa Major constellation. The North Star is itself part of the constellation of Ursa Minor.

You can gain a rough idea of your latitude by measuring the angle of the North Star over the horizon. It is no substitute, of course, for a sextant and navigational tables. Even a small margin of error in measuring the angle could put you off course by several hundred miles.

In the southern hemisphere you can use the constellation known as the Southern Cross as a guide. The four brightest stars form a cross, tilting to the side. Follow the axis of the two stars that are furthest apart, and continue on an imaginary line five times the length of this axis. Where the line ends, you will find south.

Winds

Winds flow anticlockwise around areas of low pressure in the northern hemisphere and clockwise round areas of low pressure in the southern hemisphere (cyclones). Wind systems rotate anticlockwise round centres of high pressure (anticyclones).

Between latitudes 10 degrees south and 10 degrees north is an area of low pressure and hot air known as the doldrums. On the edge of the doldrums, winds rise to create towering cumulonimbus clouds and heavy rain. At latitudes 30 degrees north and 30 degrees south from the equator, there are high-pressure belts of light variable winds. The air moving from

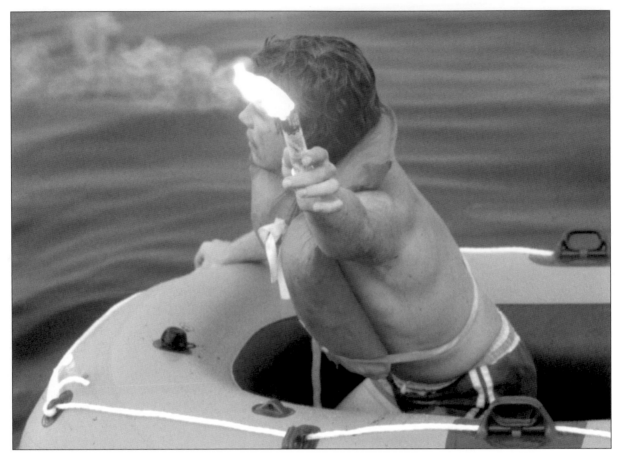

Above: In this US Army training exercise, a 'castaway' holds a flare in a life raft to attract the attention of rescuers. In a wartime scenario, the flare would be used at only the last minute, to avoid alerting the enemy.

these latitudes towards the doldrums is known as the trade winds, or the prevailing winds of the lower latitudes.

In the northern hemisphere, the prevailing wind that flows from the north southwards towards the equator is called the northeast trade wind. Deflection by the rotation of the earth means that it is not a straight north–south flow, but rather it flows diagonally, from northeast to southwest.

In the southern hemisphere, the corresponding wind is called the southeast trade wind. In the middle latitudes, the winds are called the prevailing westerlies, although their direction can be affected by a number of factors. In the summer, the land forms areas of low pressure, which attracts wind from the colder oceans. In the winter, the process is reversed.

Apart from major seasonal changes and characteristics, there are also daily changes to wind effects in the local area caused by the changes of temperature on both land and at sea. In the summer, the land tends to be warmer than the sea by day, but cooler than the sea at night. The effect of this is that, during the day, breezes flow from the sea into the land, while at night breezes tend to blow from the land out to the sea.

Endurance in the Tropics

The tropics is the area of the globe between the Tropic of Cancer (latitude 23.5 degrees north) and the Tropic of Capricorn (23.5 degrees south). The tropics receive the most direct rays from the sun and they also receive high levels of rain, with more than 1.8m (6ft) of annual precipitation.

Rainfall tends to rise with the level of elevation above the sea, and there are many mountainous areas in tropical regions. The result is an abundance of vegetation, and the most diverse

CLOUDS

If you are training with military, naval or air forces, you will develop an extreme awareness of and interest in the weather, as it will have a radical effect on how you will spend your day. The best way to prepare for whatever the weather is going to throw at you is to recognize the signs. Clouds are a good way of reading the weather. Although clouds are often associated with rain or snow, this is not always the case – certain types of cloud formation mean that good weather is on the way. Clouds can generally be categorized as high, middle and low altitude, taking the measurement between the ground and the base of the cloud.

HIGH CLOUDS (5000M; 16,500 FEET)
● Cirrus: these clouds occur at about 6km (4 miles) above the ground and are composed of ice particles. They look feathery and elongated, and are collected in bands, known as mare's tails. Although these clouds are often an indication of good weather, if they are accompanied by a north wind in cold climates they can also signal a blizzard.

● Cirrostratus: these clouds appear as a fine, hazy veil and sometimes produce a halo effect. If they accompany cirrus clouds, bad weather may be approaching.

● Cirrocumulus: these small balls of white cloud at high altitude are a cheering sight, as they are usually a sign of good weather.

MIDDLE CLOUDS (2000–5000M; 6500–16,500FT)
● Altostratus: these clouds are generally grey or blue, and they are associated with rain or snow. They can be dangerous for aircraft, as ice can gather on an airframe.

● Altocumulus: these clouds have the appearance of cotton wool, occurring either in balls or in longer fleecy strands.

LOW CLOUDS (2000M; 6500FT)
● Stratus: these low, grey clouds almost invariably mean either rain or snow.

● Nimbostratus: low, grey and often dark clouds, these occur in layers that presage rain, snow or sleet.

● Stratocumulus: these large, dark clouds with rounded tops occur in waves or lines.

● Cumulonimbus: this is a dense cloud that rises to a great height. As its appearance suggests, anything that comes out of it will be heavy, including rain, thunderstorms and snow.

vegetation types in the world, as well as the greatest diversity of animal life on the planet.

The temperature is generally high in the tropics and fairly constant due to the relative lack of wind. This is because the forest canopy filters sunlight and limits wind movement.

The forest canopy has three main layers:
1) the canopy;
2) shrubs, young trees, herbs and lianas;
3) tree branches, twigs and foliage.

The forest floor is made up of humus and fallen leaves.

Monsoon Forest

Made up of deciduous trees that shed their leaves in the dry season, this type of forest is largely found in the jungles of Southeast Asia, especially Burma, Thailand, Indonesia and Malaysia. Typical vegetation includes tall teak trees and bamboo thickets.

Mangrove Swamps

These areas can be found in both tropical and subtropical regions, including the river deltas of the Amazon, Mekong, Congo and Ganges rivers. They are characterized by dangerous animals, such as crocodiles and alligators, as well as leeches and stinging insects.

Freshwater Swamps

These swamps are normally located near rivers that supply them with water. The water flows through thick vegetation which may include palm trees and sedges. It is easy to conceal yourself in swamps, and they can be useful for surprise attacks during hunting. As some swamps are occupied by alligators or crocodiles, however, you need to be cautious about where you go.

Savanna

Savannas occur in tropical regions about 8 to 20 degrees from the equator, the most extensive being in Africa, including the Serengeti. They are generally covered with grass, with occasional woodland and shrubs. Bushfires are common. Mean annual precipitation is in the region of 80 to 150cm (31 to 59in), with rain mostly falling

SURVIVAL IN TEMPERATE FORESTS

Although temperate forests do not present the extremes of temperature that can be found in desert or arctic environments, depending on the season you can still suffer severely from cold or poor nutrition if you do not provide yourself with shelter, food and warmth.

You can build yourself a simple lean-to shelter with cut branches or, especially if there is danger of the ground becoming wet, take the time to construct a platform shelter. There is a variety of types of fire that can be built, including the safety night fire, the long fire, the star fire and the pyramid fire.

A variety of traps can be constructed to catch animals, and you can also set lines for fish. All the techniques required for these aspects of survival will either be derived from professional training or from a good training manual. It is extremely important to carry with you a good survival kit, which will provide you with all of the essentials for making fires and trapping, along with instructions.

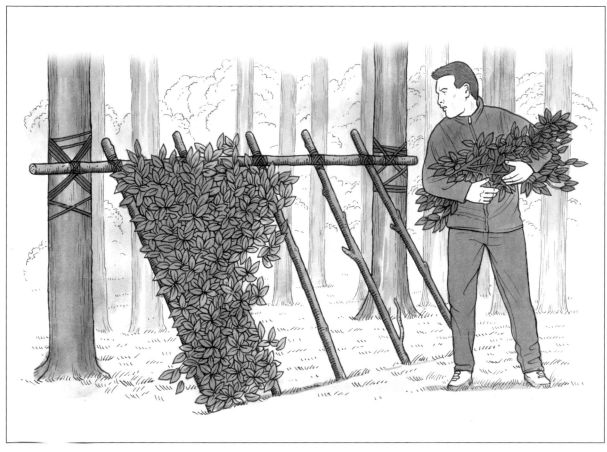

Above: Developing skills in building a simple shelter such as a lean-to can make a huge difference, either on regular exercises or on escape-and-evasion. The choice of shelter will depend on the materials available.

between October and March in the southern hemisphere and between April and September in the northern hemisphere. Mean monthly temperatures are between 10°C (50°F) and 20°C (68°F) in the dry season and 20°C (68°F) and 30°C (86°F) in the wet season.

Clothing in the Tropics

If you are in the jungle, you will need thorn-proof clothing, as well as boots that are strong and breathable. Jungle boots are often fitted with a metal plate to prevent any sharp objects from penetrating through the sole of the boot and into your foot. You will need to change your socks as often as possible. One way of getting a damp pair to dry is to tie them round your waist. Due to the humidity your clothing will almost inevitably become soaked with sweat. In order to get a comfortable night's sleep, put on your spare dry clothes at night, then put your damp clothes back on in the morning. You should powder your body with zinc talcum powder and use insect repellent.

Movement in the Jungle

Jungle travel can be very awkward, not only because of the often dense vegetation, but also because it is difficult to take bearings due

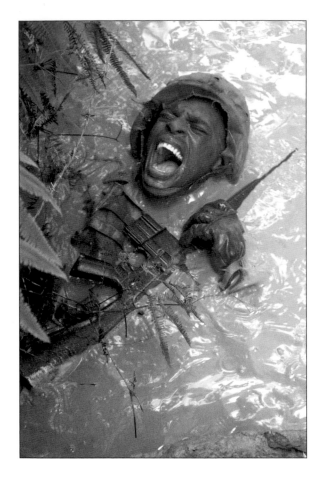

and on different gradients. For example, you should know your pace for climbing a hill as opposed to walking on the flat. If you are in a tropical area, work out different paces for swamp, jungle, savanna, and so on.

Trails and river courses may be used by enemy soldiers and dangerous animals at night, and jungle trails can be treacherous and confusing. If you are in a hostile environment, the trails could well be booby trapped. Trails in jungles tend to follow the contours of the land, along valleys or along ridges. If you head straight across country, you will probably travel at no more than 0.6km/h (1mph) and probably no more than 5km (3 miles) in a day, taking everything into consideration.

You should avoid mangrove swamps if possible, as they are extremely difficult to navigate and you may find yourself having to turn back or getting into some difficulty. On dry land, beware of areas in gullies where broken trees and branches may have accumulated, disguised by a layer of moss. You can fall right through the vegetation and sustain an injury.

To cross streams and rivers, you may attempt a river crossing or make a raft out of bamboo. If so, you will need to keep an eye out for dangerous animals such as crocodiles, caimans or alligators. You should regularly remove leeches and attend to any scratches or grazes immediately, lest they become infected.

When choosing a place to camp, select a site with solid ground away from insects and from any rotting branches or other overhead dangers. Although very hot and sultry by day, the jungle can be very cold at night, so make sure your bed

to the thick jungle canopy. Jungle paths can be bewildering and deceptive, and you could soon find yourself going round in circles. One navigation option is to take a bearing on a point that you can keep in sight, and once you have reached it take another bearing. It can be difficult in the jungle, however, to distinguish one point from another due to the density of foliage. If you are in a group, you can get one person to move to a desired point in your line of march, then move to that point, before getting him to move on again.

You should learn to pace in order to measure the distance travelled. Trained soldiers will have learned their own stride lengths and should have recorded their paces in different environments is dry and that you are nowhere near any water that is likely to seep into your camp. Ideally you should be in a hammock slung between two trees, if you are carrying the right equipment.

Endurance in Mountains

Major mountain systems are to be found across the world, including the Rocky Mountains of northwestern North America, the Andes on the west coast of South America, the Sierra Nevada and the Appalachians. The Eurasian mountain system includes the Pyrenees mountains, separating France and Spain, the Alps, the Carpathians, the Urals and, of course, the Hindu Kush and the Himalaya. In North Africa, there are the Atlas mountains and in Australia the Great Dividing Range.

Mountain Climate

The temperature falls at a rate of about 0.5° to 1°C for every 100m (328ft). Rainfall is higher on the windward slopes due to the effect of the wind being forced upwards and then cooling. Once the wind has gone over the top of the hill, it then descends down the leeward slope, warming up as it goes. This creates a rain-shadow effect.

Desert mountains, however, experience little rain, due to the dry nature of the air. Equatorial mountains have no seasonal changes, but there are rapid changes in temperature, from about –2°C (28°F) to 8°C (46°F). Mountainsides in temperate regions that face the equator are considerably warmer than mountainsides facing away from the equator.

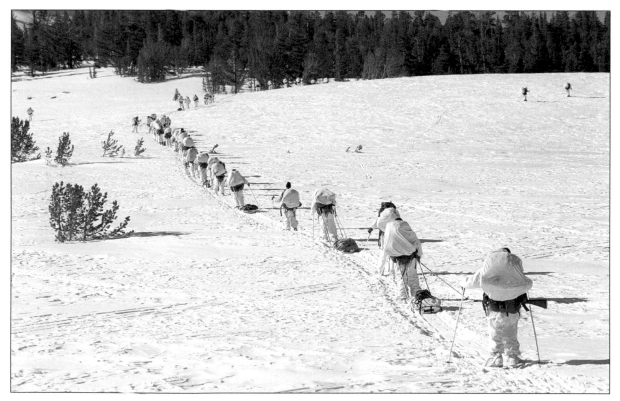

Above: A US mountain regiment moves across snow in Bridgeport, California, pulling heavy loads. Cold weather and arctic survival traning is essential for preparing troops for every type of environment.

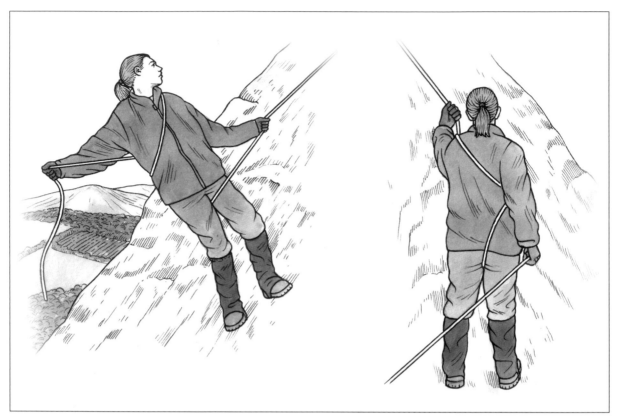

Above: Rappelling should be practised only under supervision or after training. The rope is first tied securely to one or more anchors, a knot is made at the other end, then it is passed from front to rear, round the upper left thigh, diagonally across the chest, over the right shoulder, under the armpit and into the left hand.

Mountain ranges close to the coast have a maritime climate that is generally mild, but which produces more rain and snow. Further inland, the temperatures become more extreme, with very cold winters and very hot summers. Whatever the climate, the weather on mountains can change quickly and unpredictably, which means that you have to carry suitable equipment and clothing at all times. Due to the lack of vegetation at greater heights, there is little natural protection from wind and rain.

The speed and force of the wind increases as you go higher. As the wind runs off hard surfaces, it may be funnelled in unpredictable ways that can catch you off guard. With wind comes the wind-chill factor. The natural temperature in a calm environment can fall by the equivalent of more than 50 per cent due to the effects of wind chill in a wind speed of around 19km/h (12mph). Snow is unpredictable and can fall in any season at heights of more than 1500m (5000ft). Fresh falls of snow also increase the likelihood of avalanches and may radically change the appearance of the landscape, causing disorientation.

As you approach a mountain, you will typically pass through deciduous broad-leaved forests, then an evergreen coniferous forest, before you reach what is known as the timberline. The timberline is the area above which photosynthesis

PRINCIPLES OF MILITARY CLIMBING

The basic principle of climbing is that the weight should be centred over the feet while the hands are used mostly for balance.

For military units, a climb is normally part of a tactical manoeuvre to surprise and enemy, although this may not always be the quickest and easiest route. The principles of climbing involve the smooth transition of weight from one point of the body to another based on five body parts, namely the trunk of the body, the two hands and the two feet. Only one of the five body parts is moved at any one time.

In the correct climbing position, the climber is balanced over both feet, with legs kept straight. If the climber is too close to the rock, the weight tends to force the climber's feet away from the rock. The arms should not be stretched up the rock surface, but kept in an area roughly between waist and shoulder. Three points of contact should ideally be maintained at all times, which may mean the weight resting on one foot with the hands on two hand holds.

When moving, shift the weight on to one foot and move the other foot to a new position, which should not alter your body position or balance. Restore balance on both feet, then shift weight on to the recently moved foot so that the other foot can be moved. Restore balance on both feet, then move one hand to an area between waist and head height. Then move the other hand.

To maximize friction on the rock with both feet, you should aim for maximum sole contact, ideally with the entire boot. This should also provide maximum rest for your legs. Avoid the temptation to place weight on your arms and hands. Handholds should be used to keep the climber into the face of the rock and not for bearing weight. All holds should be tested before weight is committed to them.

SOME PRINCIPAL WORLD MOUNTAINS:

Mountain	Height	Location
Mount Elbert	4401m (14,438ft)	Rocky Mountains, Colorado
Mount Logan	5959m (19,550ft)	Canada
Mount McKinley	6194m (20,321ft)	Canada
Pico de Orizaba	5610m (18,405ft)	Mexico
Popocatpetl	5465m (17,929ft)	Mexico
Mount Whitney	4421m (14,504ft)	Sierra Nevada
Aconcagua	6962m (22,841ft)	Argentina
Huascaran	6768m (22,204ft)	Peru
Ojos de Salado	6887m (22,560ft)	Chile
Cerro de Torre	6168m (20,236ft)	Patagonia
Mount Chimborazo	6310m (20,700ft)	Ecuador
Atlas Toubkal	4165m (13,664ft)	Morocco
Mount Kenya	5195m (17,043ft)	Kenya
Kilimanjaro	5895m (19,340ft)	Kenya/Tanzania

RAPPELLING

Rappelling is a technique which is used for quick descents.

● Install primary and secondary anchors above the level of the start of the rappel.

● Always wear gloves.

● The feet should be shoulder-width apart, legs and back straight. When carrying equipment, the legs should be lower than the buttocks to compensate for the extra weight.

● The rappeller looks over the brake shoulder.

● The guide arm is locked, with elbow extended; the rope is allowed to slide through the guide hand.

● The rate of descent is regulated by the brake hand.

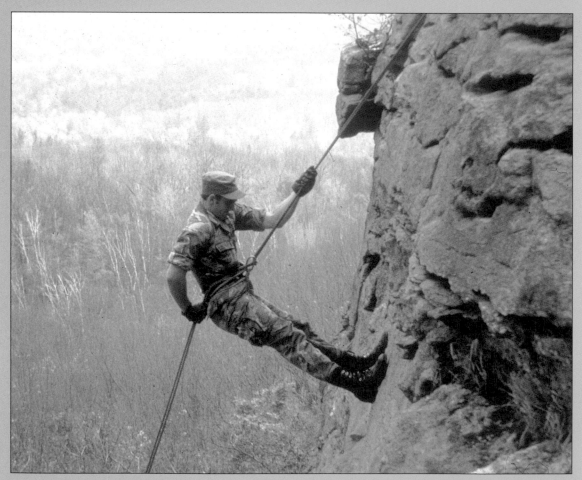

Above: A member of the US Marine Corps demonstrates correct rappelling technique. Note that gloves are worn and that the feet are evenly spread.

is not strong enough for trees to grow. From this point you will find tundra-like dwarf shrubs and herbs. There may be grass on some slopes, arranged in tussocks.

As you move on upwards, vegetation may disappear altogether. Rocks tend to fall down from the higher areas, and these will collect on flatter ground. Smaller stone slopes are known as scree slopes, and they can be difficult to negotiate on an upward climb because of the slippery nature of the ground. Snow cover presents its own challenges and advantages. The cover may be too deep to traverse in some places, but it may also smooth over otherwise difficult terrain.

Endurance Training in Mountains

The phrase 'It's tough at the top' has a particular relevance to military mountain training. It is true that soldiers have to survive against the elements whenever they are outdoors; however, in a mountain environment, many environmental difficulties are exacerbated.

The utilization of water by the body is increased in a mountain environment due to the relatively dry air that is taken into the lungs. This means that additional water supplies must be carried. High altitudes also mean there is a lack of oxygen, which can lead to altitude sickness and decreased mental performance. The range of mountain sickness may include acute mountain sickness (AMS), high-altitude pulmonary edema (HAPE) or high-altitude cerebral edema (HACE).

The best way to reduce the risk of suffering mountain sickness is through the process of acclimatization. An ascent should be made to a moderate altitude and a pause allowed for about three days before moving on to the next level. A similar effect can be achieved by a graded ascent, whereby each night's sleep is only about

BELAY TECHNIQUES

Belaying is a technique whereby the climber manages the rope in such a way as to be able to arrest a fall by another climber: this is normally achieved by applying a brake in case of a potential fall.

● The belayer needs to be aware of the terrain to be able to use it to its best advantage.

● The belayer should be able to brace himself, preferably in a sitting position, and be prepared to take the strain from a number of angles.

● There should be at least two anchors for a downward pull.

● Anchor attachments and rope should be on the side of the guide hand.

● Always keep the brake hand on the rope.

● Call 'Belay in!' when everything is ready.

● Maintain the belay at all times until the climber calls 'Belay off!'

91m (300ft) above the altitude of the previous night's sleep.

Depending on the height and severity of the weather, soldiers may suffer a wide range of cold-associated injuries, including frostbite, hypothermia, trench foot and snow blindness. It is extremely important, therefore, to both wear and carry the correct equipment, including a layered clothing system, headwear, protective goggles and boots.

As with those who take on a new sport, a new set of muscles will be used by those in mountain environments, which call for constant balance work at angles, ascents and descents, and a wide range of upper-body and arm work. The

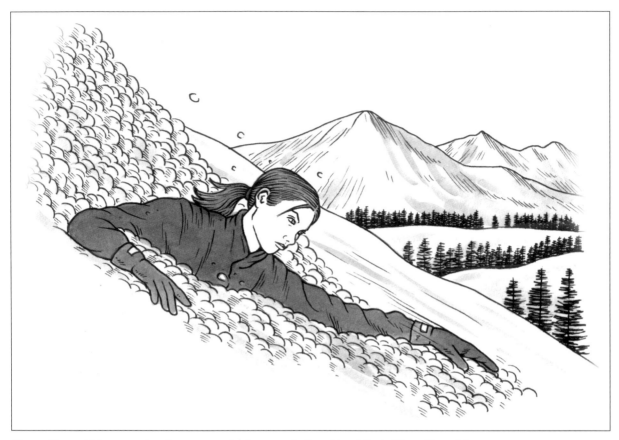

Above: If caught by an avalanche, you can try to move to the side of the fall by rolling sideways, or you can use swimming motions to try to remain close to the surface and so ride out the avalanche. If under the snow, clear a breathing space in front of the face, as the possibility of suffocation is acute.

MOVEMENT ON SNOW AND ICE

- Use either or both an ice axe or crampons.
- On traversing moderate slopes, the ice axe is held by the head on the up-slope side of the body and the pick facing the rear.
- On steeper slopes, hold the ice axe across the body with the spike into the hill. The pick points to the rear.
- On very steep slopes, drive the pick into the slope, holding it at the shaft; alternatively drive the pick into the ice, holding it by the head, like a dagger.
- Crampons can be driven into the ice using the toe of the boot, and weight gradually distributed on to the spikes at the front of the boot.
- When traversing on crampons, keep the crampons flat on the surface, stamping if necessary to gain purchase on the ice.

greater your cardiovascular (aerobic) endurance, the better you will be able to cope with the extreme physical exertion in areas where there is little oxygen. There is no substitute for actual physical training in the actual environment. In other words, if you are planning to do mountain work, you will benefit from doing a wide range of hill walking and scrambling, with increased loads on your back as you grow fitter. You should also, of course, build in some actual climbing work.

Weight training will strengthen all of your body muscles, and if you are a runner with good leg strength it will develop your upper body and arms to provide the strength you need for climbing. Swimming will help to improve your

MOVEMENT IN MOUNTAINS

Adhere to the following rules when moving in mountainous terrain:
● At all times strive to retain your balance, with your weight centred over your feet.
● Take moderate steps, straightening the knee after each movement.
● If moving in a group, or roped together, an agreed space should be maintained between individuals to allow for differences of pace, according to terrain.
● Keep a regular pace, allowing reasonable time for rest, ideally on level ground.
● On extreme inclines, the rest-step can be employed: after each step forward, lock your rear leg and shift your weight on it.
● Avoid walking along the side of hills where possible, especially when carrying weights on your back.

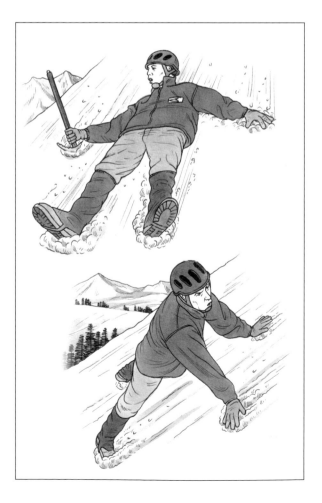

lung capacity, which is an important consideration in areas with low oxygen.

Mental endurance is required to maintain personal and operational effectiveness in an extremely rugged and challenging environment. The vast proportion of mountain work requires some form of risk, as well as acute physical demands. Elite forces involved in mountain work are taught a high level of self-reliance as well as the ability to work successfully in a small team in order to provide the best chance of survival.

Left: A mountaineer can break a fall by spreading his or her arms and legs, and creating the maximum amount of friction and drag.

Index

PICTURE CREDITS